Sniper NEET PG Vol. 1

PSM, Pathology & Microbiology – 10 Years Recall + Ultrafast Revision MCQs

Dr (Major) Debasish Das
MBBS (Trivandrum), MD (Army Hospital R&R, New Delhi)
Consultant Anesthesiologist
Assam Cancer Care Foundation

ISBN: 978-93-342-8357-0

First Edition: 2025
Published by: Dr Debasish Das

This book is intended as a quick reference and rapid review tool for NEET PG aspirants. It does not replace in-depth subject reading, clinical experience, or standard academic sources.

"For my parents — who saw the dream in me before I could."

Preface

This book is designed as a sniper-style rapid revision tool for NEET PG aspirants. It includes ten years of previous year questions, classified facts, tables, and recall-based sections in PSM, Pathology, and Microbiology. The focus is sharp and concise—to help you revise in the final few days with utmost clarity and confidence.

About the Author

Dr (Major) Debasish Das is a Consultant Anesthesiologist at Assam Cancer Care Foundation. He earned his MBBS from Medical College Trivandrum (Kerala University) and completed his MD in Anesthesiology from Army Hospital Research & Referral, New Delhi (Delhi University).

With over 20 years of service across diverse sectors—from medical colleges and government hospitals (teaching and non-teaching) to military establishments and corporate hospitals—he has mentored countless young doctors across India.

Through these years, he observed a recurring pattern: a significant number of junior doctors struggling to balance clinical duties and NEET PG preparation. Many lacked access to proper mentorship and sharp, focused revision tools. Most importantly, they yearned for a rapid-fire question bank of past-year MCQs that could be completed in just a week—without disrupting their already overwhelmed schedules.

This book is a response to that need. Designed as a killer, ultra-concentrated, last-minute revision tool, it's made to boost your chances without burning you out.

"I've seen the struggle firsthand. This book is your sniper scope in the chaos — to help you aim, fire, and succeed."

— Dr (Major) Debasish Das

How to Use This Book Efficiently

This book is designed as a rapid revision weapon, not a textbook. The goal is to help you recall maximum facts with minimum effort in the final lap of NEET PG prep.

🔷 1. Start with the Bonus Sections
They contain recall-style, high-yield questions to test your readiness. Use them as a warm-up or rapid-fire drill before each subject.

🔷 2. Use the Rapidfire One-Liners Daily
Glance through 10–15 pages daily. These are curated from PYQs and standard references and are gold for last-minute memory anchoring.

🔷 3. Visual Tables & Charts = Better Retention
Pathology and Microbiology are heavy on facts. Use the visual summaries and classification charts to cut through the clutter.

🔷 4. Flip Through Sections Randomly
You don't need to go in order. This book is meant for repeated revision in short bursts. Flip, recall, and reinforce.

🔷 5. Focus on Pattern Recognition
Many MCQs are based on recurring themes. As you revise, train your brain to identify repetitive question styles.

🔷 6. No Time? Just the Bold Parts. On days you feel overwhelmed, just revise the bold points or tables. That alone will give you 60–70% strike power.

Use this book like a sniper rifle, not a machine gun. Precise, powerful, and purposeful.

Contents

NEET PG PSM PYQs

Q1. A 52-year-old woman with no complaints comes for a routine check-up. What is the level of prevention involved?
◦ A. Primordial ◦ B. Primary ◦ C. Secondary◦ D. Tertiary

✅ **Ans:** C. Secondary

Explanation:
Secondary prevention = **early detection** in asymptomatic stage to reduce disease impact (e.g., screening tests, mammography, Pap smear).

Topic insight:
Primary = prevent disease onset (vaccination, lifestyle)
Secondary = early detection (screening)
Tertiary = rehabilitation
Primordial = prevent risk factor emergence (urban planning, health education)

Q2. A newborn receives OPV at birth. This is an example of which type of vaccine?
◦ A. Killed vaccine
◦ B. Toxoid
◦ C. Live attenuated vaccine
◦ D. Subunit vaccine

✅ **Ans:** C. Live attenuated vaccine

Explanation:
OPV (Oral Polio Vaccine – Sabin) contains **live, weakened virus** that replicates in the gut and induces mucosal & systemic immunity.

Topic insight:
Live vaccines: OPV, BCG, MMR, yellow fever
Killed: IPV, Hep A
Subunit: Hep B, HPV
Toxoid: Tetanus, Diphtheria

Q3. What is the most sensitive indicator of health status of a community?
◦ A. Infant mortality rate (IMR)
◦ B. Perinatal mortality rate
◦ C. Crude death rate
◦ D. Life expectancy

✅ **Ans:** A. Infant mortality rate

Explanation:
IMR = number of infant deaths (<1 year) per 1000 live births → reflects **healthcare, nutrition, sanitation, and maternal care**.

Topic insight:
IMR is sensitive to **both prenatal and postnatal** care
Lower IMR = better public health system

Q4. The prevalence of hypertension in a city is found to be 15%. What does it reflect?
◦ A. Incidence
◦ B. Risk
◦ C. Burden
◦ D. Mortality

✅ **Ans:** C. Burden

Explanation:
Prevalence measures **existing cases** (old + new) → indicates disease **burden** in the community at a given point.

Topic insight:
Prevalence = Incidence × Duration
Chronic diseases → high prevalence, low incidence
Acute diseases → high incidence, low prevalence

Q5. What is the denominator in Crude Birth Rate (CBR)?
◦ A. Population at risk
◦ B. Mid-year population
◦ C. Total number of births
◦ D. Number of married women
✅ **Ans:** B. Mid-year population
Explanation:
CBR = (Total live births in 1 year / Mid-year population) × 1000
Topic insight:
Mid-year population ≈ population on July 1st
CBR reflects fertility & reproductive health services

Q6. Which of the following is an example of herd immunity?
◦ A. Immunity after infection
◦ B. Community protection from measles due to MMR vaccine
◦ C. Maternal IgG crossing placenta
◦ D. Hepatitis B immunoglobulin
✅ **Ans:** B. Community protection from measles due to MMR vaccine
Explanation:
Herd immunity = when **enough people are immune**, even unvaccinated individuals are protected due to **reduced transmission**.
Topic insight:
Works only for **communicable** diseases
Does NOT protect against **tetanus**, which is non-contagious

---

Q7. A 3-year-old child with no past immunizations comes for the first dose of DPT. Which schedule is followed?
◦ A. 0, 6, 10 weeks
◦ B. 6, 10, 14 weeks
◦ C. 9 months, 16 months
◦ D. 5 years and 10 years
✅ **Ans:** B. 6, 10, 14 weeks
Explanation:
DPT1–3 given at 6, 10, 14 weeks under **National Immunization Schedule**.
Topic insight:
DPT booster at **16–24 months** and **5 years**
DTaP for fewer side effects (in private sector)

Q8. In a screening test, what does a high sensitivity imply?
◦ A. Fewer false positives
◦ B. Fewer false negatives
◦ C. Higher prevalence
◦ D. Greater specificity
✅ **Ans:** B. Fewer false negatives
Explanation:
Sensitivity = ability to **detect true positives**
High sensitivity → low **false negatives** → useful in **screening tests**
Topic insight:
SNOUT: SeNsitive test when Negative rules OUT disease
SPIN: SPecific test when Positive rules IN disease

Q9. An index case of measles is isolated. What type of prevention is this?
◦ A. Primary
◦ B. Secondary

◦ C. Tertiary
◦ D. Primordial

✅ **Ans:** A. Primary

Explanation:
Primary prevention = **preventing spread or occurrence** of disease in contacts via **isolation, vaccination, health education**

Topic insight:
Isolation = infected person
Quarantine = healthy exposed person

Q10. A community health worker administers TT to a pregnant woman. What type of prevention is this?
◦ A. Primary
◦ B. Secondary
◦ C. Tertiary
◦ D. Primordial

✅ **Ans:** A. Primary

Explanation:
Vaccination is **primary prevention** – prevents disease onset (maternal & neonatal tetanus in this case)

Q11. What is the minimum coverage required to interrupt measles transmission in a population?
◦ A. 50%
◦ B. 70%
◦ C. 85%
◦ D. 95%

✅ **Ans:** D. 95%

Explanation:
Measles has a **very high R_0 (~15–18)**. Hence, **≥95% vaccine coverage** is required to achieve herd immunity and interrupt transmission.

Topic insight:
Higher R_0 → higher herd immunity threshold
Measles elimination = ≥95% coverage + strong surveillance

Q12. Which of the following is the correct sequence in levels of health care in India?
◦ A. Subcenter → PHC → CHC → District hospital
◦ B. PHC → Subcenter → CHC → District hospital
◦ C. CHC → PHC → Subcenter → District hospital
◦ D. District hospital → CHC → PHC → Subcenter

✅ **Ans:** A. Subcenter → PHC → CHC → District hospital

Explanation:
This is the **referral hierarchy** under rural health infrastructure.

Topic insight:
Subcenter = first contact in rural areas
PHC = for ~30,000 people
CHC = referral unit for 4 PHCs (1:1,20,000 population)
DH = full-fledged secondary care

Q13. What is the main objective of ASHA (Accredited Social Health Activist)?
◦ A. Conducting deliveries
◦ B. Providing medicine at village level
◦ C. Health awareness & linkage to services
◦ D. Handling emergencies

✅ **Ans:** C. Health awareness & linkage to services

Explanation:
ASHA = bridge between community and health system under **NRHM** (2005). She is trained to **mobilize**, counsel, and support basic care.

Topic insight:
1 ASHA/1000 rural population
Not a provider but a **facilitator**

Q14. Which of the following is a health promotion strategy?
◦ A. Screening for breast cancer
◦ B. Isolation of cases
◦ C. Dietary counseling for obesity
◦ D. Antibiotics for TB
✅ **Ans:** C. Dietary counseling for obesity
Explanation:
Health promotion includes **behavioral modification, lifestyle change**, and empowerment for well-being – not treatment or diagnosis.
Topic insight:
Ottawa Charter: 5 components of health promotion
Counseling, education, policy change = health promotion

Q15. A diagnostic test has low sensitivity and high specificity. Which is most likely to happen?
◦ A. High false positives
◦ B. High false negatives
◦ C. No error
◦ D. High true positives
✅ **Ans:** B. High false negatives
Explanation:
Low sensitivity = more **false negatives** (disease present but test misses). High specificity → fewer false positives.
Topic insight:
Screening: prioritize **sensitivity**
Confirmation: prioritize **specificity**

Q16. Which is the first step in outbreak investigation?
◦ A. Descriptive epidemiology
◦ B. Confirm the outbreak
◦ C. Develop hypothesis
◦ D. Verify diagnosis
✅ **Ans:** D. Verify diagnosis
Explanation:
Before calling it an outbreak, you must **confirm diagnosis** to rule out misreporting or lab error.
Topic insight (Epidemiology Steps):
Prepare
Confirm diagnosis
Confirm outbreak
Define case
Descriptive study
Develop/test hypothesis
Control
Report

Q17. A disease has high case fatality rate (CFR). What does this indicate?
◦ A. High infectivity
◦ B. High severity
◦ C. High prevalence
◦ D. Long duration
✅ **Ans:** B. High severity
Explanation:
CFR = (deaths among cases / total cases) × 100
→ Higher CFR = **more lethal/severe disease**.
Topic insight:
Ebola, rabies → high CFR
Common cold → low CFR

Q18. Which of the following is NOT included in the demographic cycle?
◦ A. Late expanding
◦ B. Early expanding
◦ C. Stationary
◦ D. Sustainablc

✅ **Ans:** D. Sustainable
Explanation:
"Sustainable" is not a demographic phase. There are **5 standard stages** of demographic cycle.
Topic insight (Demographic Cycle):
High stationary
Early expanding
Late expanding
Low stationary
Declining
India is in **Stage 3 – Late expanding**

Q19. What is the time period of infant mortality rate (IMR)?
◦ A. <1 month
◦ B. <6 months
◦ C. <1 year
◦ D. <5 years
✅ **Ans:** C. <1 year
Explanation:
IMR = **deaths of infants (<1 year)** per 1000 live births.
Topic breakdown:
Neonatal mortality = <28 days
Post-neonatal = 28 days to 1 year
Under-5 mortality = <5 years

Q20. A study divides participants based on exposure and follows them over time. Type of study?
◦ A. Case-control
◦ B. Cohort
◦ C. Cross-sectional
◦ D. Experimental
✅ **Ans:** B. Cohort
Explanation:
Cohort = **exposure → outcome**
Follows groups **forward in time**, can measure **incidence and risk**
Topic insight:
Case-control = outcome → back to exposure
Cross-sectional = snapshot
Experimental = randomized trial

Q21. Which of the following vaccines is stored at sub-zero temperature?
◦ A. DPT
◦ B. TT
◦ C. BCG
◦ D. OPV
✅ **Ans:** D. OPV
Explanation:
Oral Polio Vaccine is stored at **−20°C** in deep freezers because it's **live attenuated** and highly heat sensitive.
Key tip:
OPV, Measles, BCG → sensitive to heat & light
Stored in **deep freezer**
DPT, TT → stored at **2–8°C** → freeze-sensitive

Q22. Which phase of clinical trial detects rare side effects?
◦ A. Phase I
◦ B. Phase II
◦ C. Phase III
◦ D. Phase IV
✅ **Ans:** D. Phase IV
Explanation:
Phase IV = **Post-marketing surveillance** → long-term & rare adverse effects
Topic insight:
Phase I: safety
Phase II: efficacy in patients
Phase III: comparison with current standard
Phase IV: **real-world usage**

Q23. Anemia Mukt Bharat covers which age group with iron and folic acid tablets (pink)?

◦ A. 1–5 years
◦ B. 5–10 years
◦ C. 10–19 years
◦ D. Pregnant women

✅ **Ans:** A. 1–5 years

Explanation:

In AMB:
6–59 months = **1 ml iron syrup (biweekly)**
5–9 years = pink tablet
10–19 years = blue tablet
Pregnant = red tablet

Q24. Which is the first function to be lost in cold chain breach?

◦ A. Freezing
◦ B. Thermostat control
◦ C. Heat sensitivity
◦ D. Light exposure

✅ **Ans:** C. Heat sensitivity

Explanation:

Most vaccines are **heat-sensitive**, so excess heat damages potency first.
Live vaccines (e.g., OPV) lose potency rapidly in warm climates.

Q25. An outbreak occurs in a closed community. Everyone exposed becomes symptomatic within 48 hours. Likely epidemic curve?

◦ A. Propagated
◦ B. Point source
◦ C. Continuous
◦ D. Slow epidemic

✅ **Ans:** B. Point source

Explanation:

Point source epidemic = single common exposure → rapid peak, rapid decline
(e.g., food poisoning at a wedding)

Topic contrast:

Propagated = person-to-person (e.g., measles)
Continuous = repeated exposure (e.g., polluted water)

Q26. Which program under NHM provides cash incentives for institutional deliveries?

◦ A. RCH-II
◦ B. JSY
◦ C. RMNCH+A
◦ D. PMSMA

✅ **Ans:** B. Janani Suraksha Yojana (JSY)

Explanation:

JSY provides cash to promote **safe institutional deliveries** in BPL/SC/ST women
(launched 2005 under NRHM)

Topic bonus:

JSY = cash incentive
JSSK = free transport, diet, drugs

Q27. Which color code bin is used for discarded vaccine vials?

◦ A. Yellow
◦ B. Red
◦ C. White (translucent)
◦ D. Blue

✅ **Ans:** C. White (translucent)

Explanation:

Puncture-proof white bins are for **sharps & vials** (needles, broken ampoules, empty vials)

BMW Rules 2016 quick recap:

Yellow = anatomical, infectious waste
Red = tubing, gloves, IV set
White = sharps

Blue = glass, vials

Q28. What is the mode of transmission of Q fever?
◦ A. Tick bite
◦ B. Aerosol from animal waste
◦ C. Milk ingestion
◦ D. Dog scratch
✅ **Ans:** B. Aerosol from animal waste
Explanation:
Coxiella burnetii – airborne from sheep/goat/cattle waste → highly infectious
No vector required.

Q29. How many ASHA workers are appointed per rural population?
◦ A. 1 per 500
◦ B. 1 per 1000
◦ C. 1 per 5000
◦ D. 1 per 10,000
✅ **Ans:** B. 1 per 1000
Explanation:
ASHA = Accredited Social Health Activist
1 per 1000 **rural** population; no fixed for urban.

Q30. A vaccine is given to a patient who has already been exposed to the disease. This is:
◦ A. Primary prevention
◦ B. Secondary prevention
◦ C. Tertiary prevention
◦ D. Primordial prevention
✅ **Ans:** B. Secondary prevention
Explanation:
Post-exposure prophylaxis (like **anti-rabies vaccine, Hep B vaccine**) aims to **limit disease progression**, not prevent exposure.

Q31. Which vitamin is administered to newborns to prevent hemorrhagic disease?
◦ A. Vitamin D
◦ B. Vitamin A
◦ C. Vitamin K
◦ D. Vitamin E
✅ **Ans:** C. Vitamin K
Explanation:
Vitamin K prevents **hemorrhagic disease of newborn (HDN)** caused by physiologic deficiency due to sterile gut and immature liver.
Topic bonus:
Given **IM within 1 hour of birth**
Prevents **intracranial and GI bleeds**

Q32. Which of the following is a vector for Kala-azar (Visceral leishmaniasis)?
◦ A. Anopheles
◦ B. Culex
◦ C. Phlebotomus
◦ D. Aedes
✅ **Ans:** C. Phlebotomus
Explanation:
Phlebotomus argentipes (female sandfly) transmits **Leishmania donovani**.
Topic tip:
Nocturnal biter
Control via **DDT spray**, insecticide-treated nets

Q33. Which of the following indicators is NOT included in HDI (Human Development Index)?
◦ A. Education
◦ B. Life expectancy
◦ C. Per capita income
◦ D. Infant mortality rate

✅ **Ans:** D. Infant mortality rate

Explanation:

HDI = Life expectancy + Mean years of schooling + GNI per capita

Topic insight:

IMR is used in **Physical Quality of Life Index (PQLI)**, not HDI

HDI ≠ a health-only index → composite development measure

Q34. Which is the target of "TB elimination in India" per National Strategic Plan (NSP)?

◦ A. 2022
◦ B. 2023
◦ C. 2025
◦ D. 2030

✅ **Ans:** C. 2025

Explanation:

India aims to eliminate TB **5 years before global target** (SDG = 2030).
NSP 2017–2025 outlines this goal.

Q35. Which is the most important factor for long-term health improvement in population?

◦ A. Immunization
◦ B. Housing
◦ C. Nutrition
◦ D. Literacy

✅ **Ans:** D. Literacy

Explanation:

Literacy (especially female literacy) impacts fertility, nutrition, health-seeking behavior and long-term well-being.

Bonus clue:

Often tested as "social determinant" of health

Education → empowerment → better choices

Q36. What is the unit of measurement in Sullivan's index?

◦ A. Quality-adjusted life years (QALY)
◦ B. Disability-adjusted life years (DALY)
◦ C. Expectation of life free of disability
◦ D. Years of life lost

✅ **Ans:** C. Expectation of life free of disability

Explanation:

Sullivan index = **life expectancy – years lived with disability**

Used to measure **quality of health**, not just survival.

Q37. What is the incubation period of measles?

◦ A. 2–4 days
◦ B. 7–10 days
◦ C. 10–14 days
◦ D. 21 days

✅ **Ans:** C. 10–14 days

Explanation:

Measles incubation = ~**10 days to fever**, ~14 days to rash

Highly contagious: **airborne** transmission

Q38. A clinical trial assigns patients into two groups and compares outcomes. It is:

◦ A. Observational cohort
◦ B. Case-control
◦ C. Randomized controlled trial (RCT)
◦ D. Cross-sectional study

✅ **Ans:** C. Randomized controlled trial (RCT)

Explanation:

RCT = **gold standard for interventions**

Features randomization, blinding, control → **reduces bias**

Q39. A study finds that obesity and type 2 diabetes are associated. What is this called?
◦ A. Confounding
◦ B. Causation
◦ C. Correlation
◦ D. Interaction

✅ **Ans:** C. Correlation
Explanation:
Correlation = **association**, not causation
Positive correlation: both variables rise together

Q40. Which of the following is a notifiable disease in India?
◦ A. Hypertension
◦ B. Diabetes
◦ C. Tuberculosis
◦ D. Anemia

✅ **Ans:** C. Tuberculosis
Explanation:
TB made notifiable in 2012 — mandatory to report all diagnosed TB cases (private/public sector)

Q41. Which of the following indices assesses undernutrition in children <5 years?
◦ A. BMI
◦ B. Mid-upper arm circumference
◦ C. Broca's index
◦ D. Waist-hip ratio

✅ **Ans:** B. Mid-upper arm circumference (MUAC)
Explanation:
MUAC <11.5 cm in 6–59 months = **severe acute malnutrition (SAM)**
Easy, low-resource field tool by ICDS, WHO, UNICEF

Q42. Which test is used to compare means between **two independent groups**?
◦ A. Chi-square test
◦ B. t-test
◦ C. ANOVA
◦ D. Fisher's exact test

✅ **Ans:** B. t-test
Explanation:
Unpaired t-test = compare **mean of continuous variable** between **2 unrelated groups**
Extra clue:
Chi-square → categorical data
ANOVA → ≥3 groups
Fisher exact → small sample (categorical)

Q43. Which route has the **highest vaccine coverage** in India?
◦ A. Oral
◦ B. Intramuscular
◦ C. Subcutaneous
◦ D. Intradermal

✅ **Ans:** A. Oral
Explanation:
Oral Polio Vaccine (OPV) is administered orally and has widest coverage under **Universal Immunization Program (UIP)**
Bonus:
BCG → ID
MMR, JE → SC
DPT, Hep B, Pentavalent → IM

Q44. Which level of prevention includes rehabilitation for stroke survivors?

◦ A. Primordial
◦ B. Primary
◦ C. Secondary
◦ D. Tertiary

✅ **Ans:** D. Tertiary

Explanation:
Tertiary prevention = **limiting disability, restoring function**
→ Physiotherapy, occupational therapy, counseling

Q45. Which of the following diseases has a **toxoid** vaccine?
◦ A. Hepatitis B
◦ B. Tetanus
◦ C. Rabies
◦ D. Influenza

✅ **Ans:** B. Tetanus

Explanation:
Tetanus toxoid is an **inactivated bacterial exotoxin** that retains immunogenicity.
Toxoid vaccines:
Tetanus
Diphtheria
→ Given as DPT, Td, TT

Q46. A disease is present at **low constant frequency** in a region. It is called:
◦ A. Epidemic
◦ B. Sporadic
◦ C. Endemic
◦ D. Pandemic

✅ **Ans:** C. Endemic

Explanation:
Endemic = constant, predictable presence of disease in area (e.g., malaria in tribal India)

Q47. Which component of primary health care is **not included in Alma-Ata declaration**?
◦ A. Health education
◦ B. Provision of safe water
◦ C. Emergency surgery
◦ D. Immunization

✅ **Ans:** C. Emergency surgery

Explanation:
Alma Ata (1978) lists **8 essential components**, including:
Health education
Immunization
Water, sanitation
Maternal/child care
...but not surgical services

Q48. DOTS strategy is used for which disease?
◦ A. Malaria
◦ B. Tuberculosis
◦ C. AIDS
◦ D. Dengue

✅ **Ans:** B. Tuberculosis

Explanation:
Directly Observed Treatment Short-course (DOTS) is the WHO strategy for TB control under **RNTCP**

Q49. What is the surveillance type in which **all health facilities report** even when no case is found?
◦ A. Passive
◦ B. Sentinel
◦ C. Active
◦ D. Universal

✅ **Ans:** D. Universal

Explanation:
Universal surveillance = all sites must report (including "zero" reporting), e.g., polio, leprosy programs

Q50. An epidemic curve shows **gradual rise and fall** with multiple peaks. Type?
◦ A. Point source
◦ B. Propagated
◦ C. Continuous exposure
◦ D. Common source
✅ **Ans:** B. Propagated
Explanation:
Propagated outbreak = **person-to-person spread**
→ Each peak represents new generation of cases (e.g., measles, flu)

Q51. Which is the first national program launched in India?
◦ A. Malaria control
◦ B. Family planning
◦ C. Leprosy
◦ D. Tuberculosis
✅ **Ans:** B. Family planning
Explanation:
India launched the world's **first National Family Planning Program** in **1952** — aimed at population stabilization.
Key milestones:
1952 – Family planning
1958 – Malaria control
1962 – Smallpox, TB

Q52. What is the denominator of **Maternal Mortality Ratio (MMR)**?
◦ A. Total female population
◦ B. Live births
◦ C. Total births
◦ D. Pregnancies
✅ **Ans:** B. Live births
Explanation:
MMR = (Maternal deaths / Live births) × 100,000
Focuses on **risk per live birth**, not total pregnancies

Q53. Which mosquito lays eggs **singly on water surface**?
◦ A. Culex
◦ B. Anopheles
◦ C. Aedes
◦ D. Mansonia
✅ **Ans:** B. Anopheles
Explanation:
Anopheles: lays **singly**, has **boat-shaped eggs with lateral floats**
Contrast:
Culex → egg rafts
Aedes → singly but on **dry walls**
Mansonia → under floating vegetation

Q54. Which mosquito has **daytime biting** and transmits arboviruses?
◦ A. Anopheles
◦ B. Aedes aegypti
◦ C. Culex
◦ D. Mansonia
✅ **Ans:** B. Aedes aegypti
Explanation:
Aedes = vector for **Dengue, Chikungunya, Zika, Yellow fever**
Bites during **early morning & late afternoon**

Q55. What is the validity period of Yellow Fever vaccination for international travel?
◦ A. 3 years
◦ B. Lifetime
◦ C. 10 years
◦ D. 1 year
✅ **Ans:** B. Lifetime

Explanation:
As per **WHO 2016**, yellow fever vaccine provides **lifelong immunity** after a single dose.

Q56. Best indicator of **socioeconomic status** in rural India?
◦ A. Literacy
◦ B. Occupation
◦ C. Housing type
◦ D. BPL card
✅ **Ans:** D. BPL card
Explanation:
Below Poverty Line (BPL) criteria include **income, assets, caste, education** – used for public schemes.
Alternate tools:
Modified Kuppuswamy → urban
BG Prasad → per capita income

Q57. Which is a **quantitative** tool in epidemiology?
◦ A. Focus group discussion
◦ B. Interview
◦ C. Survey
◦ D. In-depth interview
✅ **Ans:** C. Survey
Explanation:
Surveys = structured, numerical data
Others are qualitative → used in **social health research**

Q58. A study shows that handwashing reduces hospital infection by 40%. What type of impact is this?
◦ A. Efficacy
◦ B. Effectiveness
◦ C. Efficiency
◦ D. Equity
✅ **Ans:** B. Effectiveness
Explanation:
Effectiveness = performance in real-world settings
Efficacy = under ideal conditions (clinical trial)

Q59. Which program provides **monthly health checkups** to school children?
◦ A. JSY
◦ B. JSSK
◦ C. RKSK
◦ D. RBSK
✅ **Ans:** D. Rashtriya Bal Swasthya Karyakram (RBSK)
Explanation:
RBSK covers children **0–18 years**, screens for **4Ds: Defects, Diseases, Deficiencies, Developmental delays**

Q60. Which of the following is a **secondary level of care**?
◦ A. Subcenter
◦ B. PHC
◦ C. CHC
◦ D. Village health hut
✅ **Ans:** C. CHC (Community Health Centre)
Explanation:
CHC = 30-bed secondary care unit, 1 per 1.2 lakh people
Offers surgical & specialist care (medicine, OBGY, etc.)

Q61. Which of the following is **NOT transmitted by Aedes mosquito**?
◦ A. Yellow fever
◦ B. Dengue
◦ C. Filariasis
◦ D. Chikungunya
✅ **Ans:** C. Filariasis
Explanation:
Filariasis is transmitted by **Culex**

(quinquefasciatus), not Aedes.
Aedes transmits:
Dengue
Zika
Yellow fever
Chikungunya

Q62. Which of the following is a **type of active surveillance**?
◦ A. Health worker visiting houses to find TB cases
◦ B. Monthly report from PHC
◦ C. Data from hospital registers
◦ D. Death certificate analysis
✅ **Ans:** A. Health worker visiting houses
Explanation:
In **active surveillance**, health personnel **actively seek cases** (e.g., during pulse polio, TB drives).
Passive = waiting for cases to be reported

Q63. A health program using WhatsApp reminders for patient follow-up is based on:
◦ A. Behavioral model
◦ B. Health belief model
◦ C. Communication model
◦ D. Ecological model
✅ **Ans:** C. Communication model
Explanation:
Sending reminders = part of **health communication** strategy — message, sender, channel, receiver, feedback.

Q64. Which vitamin supplementation is given biannually in child health programs?
◦ A. Vitamin A
◦ B. Vitamin B1
◦ C. Vitamin D
◦ D. Vitamin C
✅ **Ans:** A. Vitamin A
Explanation:
Under **RCH & UIP**, children get **9 mega doses of Vit A** (200,000 IU) every **6 months** from 9 months to 5 years.

Q65. What is the preferred treatment in mass deworming programs for children?
◦ A. Albendazole
◦ B. Metronidazole
◦ C. Ivermectin
◦ D. Mebendazole
✅ **Ans:** A. Albendazole
Explanation:
Albendazole 400 mg is given once during **National Deworming Day** (Feb & Aug) to children 1–19 years.

Q66. Which disease is associated with **secondary attack rate**?
◦ A. Genetic disorders
◦ B. Communicable diseases
◦ C. Occupational diseases
◦ D. Nutritional deficiencies
✅ **Ans:** B. Communicable diseases
Explanation:
Secondary attack rate = spread among **contacts of a primary case** → reflects **infectivity** (e.g., flu, measles)

Q67. Which index measures **obesity in children**?
◦ A. Weight-for-age
◦ B. BMI-for-age
◦ C. Height-for-age
◦ D. MUAC
✅ **Ans:** B. BMI-for-age
Explanation:

BMI-for-age plotted on **WHO Z-score charts** → used to classify obesity, overweight in 5–19 years

---

Q68. Disease surveillance is an example of which type of prevention?
◦ A. Primordial
◦ B. Primary
◦ C. Secondary
◦ D. Tertiary

✅ **Ans:** C. Secondary

Explanation:
Surveillance helps in **early detection** and **interruption of transmission**, so it's part of **secondary prevention**

Q69. Which committee first introduced **health worker for every village**?
◦ A. Bhore
◦ B. Mudaliar
◦ C. Kartar Singh
◦ D. Shrivastav

✅ **Ans:** D. Shrivastav

Explanation:
Shrivastav Committee (1975) introduced:
Community-based worker
Integration of health and medical education

Q70. A woman returns from a trip abroad. She's kept in isolation though she shows no symptoms. What is this called?
◦ A. Isolation
◦ B. Quarantine
◦ C. Segregation
◦ D. Prevention

✅ **Ans:** B. Quarantine

Explanation:
Quarantine = restriction of movement of healthy but exposed individuals
Isolation = symptomatic individuals

Q71. Which study design is best to assess **incidence**?
◦ A. Case-control
◦ B. Cross-sectional
◦ C. Cohort
◦ D. Ecological

✅ **Ans:** C. Cohort

Explanation:
Cohort = follows exposed and unexposed groups over time → allows **measurement of incidence & risk**
Case-control and cross-sectional can't do this.

Q72. A vector transmits disease **mechanically**, not biologically. Example?
◦ A. Housefly
◦ B. Aedes
◦ C. Culex
◦ D. Tsetse fly

✅ **Ans:** A. Housefly

Explanation:
Housefly transmits pathogens **passively** (on body, legs) — e.g., typhoid, cholera
Others = **biological vectors** (development of pathogen inside vector)

Q73. Which disease is targeted for **elimination by 2030** in India's health plan?
◦ A. TB
◦ B. Leprosy
◦ C. Kala-azar
◦ D. Lymphatic filariasis

✅ **Ans:** D. Lymphatic filariasis

Explanation:
Target: **Eliminate LF by 2030** using

MDA (DEC + Albendazole) + vector control
India achieved **kala-azar elimination** status in several districts already.

Q74. What is the **gold standard** test for HIV confirmation?
◦ A. ELISA
◦ B. Western blot
◦ C. PCR
◦ D. Rapid test

✅ **Ans:** B. Western blot
Explanation:
Western blot = **confirmatory**; detects specific **HIV proteins**
ELISA = screening (high sensitivity)

Q75. Which screening test shows **maximum false positives** in low-prevalence settings?
◦ A. Low sensitivity
◦ B. Low specificity
◦ C. High specificity
◦ D. High PPV

✅ **Ans:** B. Low specificity
Explanation:
Low specificity = many **false positives**
In low prevalence, even true positives are few, so false positives dominate

---

Q76. Most sensitive test to detect **subclinical iodine deficiency** in a community?
◦ A. Goiter rate
◦ B. Neonatal TSH
◦ C. Urinary iodine
◦ D. Serum T3/T4

✅ **Ans:** C. Urinary iodine
Explanation:
Urinary iodine = **current intake status**, most sensitive
100 μg/L = normal
Goiter rate = late finding

Q77. Which vaccine is given as **intradermal injection**?
◦ A. DPT
◦ B. BCG
◦ C. Hepatitis B
◦ D. OPV

✅ **Ans:** B. BCG
Explanation:
BCG is given **intradermally** at left deltoid area at birth.
Other routes:
DPT, Hep B = IM
OPV = oral

Q78. Which is **not** a feature of randomized controlled trial (RCT)?
◦ A. Blinding
◦ B. Randomization
◦ C. Observational nature
◦ D. Ethical concern

✅ **Ans:** C. Observational nature
Explanation:
RCT = **interventional** study design — researchers assign exposure
Not observational like cohort or case-control

Q79. Which disease is included under **IDSP (Integrated Disease Surveillance Program)**?
◦ A. Hypertension
◦ B. Diabetes
◦ C. Dengue
◦ D. Cancer

✅ **Ans:** C. Dengue
Explanation:
IDSP monitors **epidemic-prone**

communicable diseases (Dengue, Malaria, JE, Leptospirosis)

Q80. Which test compares **mean BP** across 3 groups?
◦ A. t-test
◦ B. Chi-square
◦ C. ANOVA
◦ D. Correlation
✅ **Ans:** C. ANOVA
Explanation:
Analysis of variance (ANOVA) is used when comparing **means among ≥3 groups**
If only 2 → use t-test

Q81. Which of the following is true about **Serial interval**?
◦ A. Time from exposure to symptoms
◦ B. Time from infection to infectivity
◦ C. Time between symptom onset in index and secondary case
◦ D. Time from diagnosis to death
✅ **Ans:** C. Time between symptom onset in index and secondary case
Explanation:
Serial interval = time between symptom onset in primary (index) case and secondary case
Helps model **infectiousness and transmission speed**
Related terms:
Incubation period = exposure to symptom onset
Generation time = infection to infection

Q82. Which disease is **non-communicable but vaccine-preventable**?
◦ A. Hepatitis B
◦ B. Polio
◦ C. Tetanus
◦ D. Typhoid
✅ **Ans:** C. Tetanus
Explanation:
Tetanus is **not spread person-to-person**, yet prevented by vaccine
Due to spores in soil → deep wounds → neurotoxin
Hence, herd immunity concept **doesn't apply**

Q83. Which of the following is **not a part of IMNCI** strategy?
◦ A. Diarrhea
◦ B. ARI
◦ C. Measles
◦ D. Typhoid
✅ **Ans:** D. Typhoid
Explanation:
IMNCI (Integrated Management of Neonatal and Childhood Illnesses) covers:
ARI, Diarrhea, Fever (malaria, measles), Malnutrition
Not typhoid or meningitis specifically

Q84.
An epidemic shows **continuous rise and fall in cases over weeks**. Most likely curve?◦ A. Point source
◦ B. Propagated
◦ C. Common source continuous
◦ D. None
✅ **Ans:** C. Common source continuous
Explanation:
Continuous exposure (e.g., contaminated water) → gradual rise/fall
Unlike point source (sharp peak), and propagated (multiple waves)

Q85. Which type of sampling gives **each individual equal chance of selection**?
◦ A. Systematic
◦ B. Stratified
◦ C. Simple random
◦ D. Cluster

✅ **Ans:** C. Simple random
Explanation:
Simple random = everyone has **equal, independent probability** of being picked
E.g., lottery method, computer randomizer

Q86. Which is the **correct sequence** of implementing health education?
◦ A. Planning → Evaluation → Implementation
◦ B. Evaluation → Planning → Implementation
◦ C. Planning → Implementation → Evaluation
◦ D. Implementation → Planning → Evaluation

✅ **Ans:** C. Planning → Implementation → Evaluation
Explanation:
Any program (including IEC/BCC) follows this 3-step flow:
Planning
Implementation
Evaluation

Q87. A study finds a **positive correlation** between sugar intake and diabetes. What does this imply?
◦ A. Causality
◦ B. Directional association
◦ C. Bias
◦ D. Confounding

✅ **Ans:** B. Directional association
Explanation:
Correlation ≠ causation, but shows association
Positive correlation → both variables increase together

Q88. What is the **basic reproductive number (R_0)** of a disease?
◦ A. Incidence per year
◦ B. Secondary cases per index
◦ C. Mortality rate
◦ D. Attack rate

✅ **Ans:** B. Secondary cases per index
Explanation:
R_0 = average number of secondary infections from one case in a fully susceptible population
E.g., Measles R_0 ~15–18 (very high), COVID ~2–3 (variable)

Q89. Which study design is best for **rare diseases**?
◦ A. Cohort
◦ B. Case-control
◦ C. Cross-sectional
◦ D. RCT

✅ **Ans:** B. Case-control
Explanation:
In rare disease: start from **cases → find exposures (retrospective)**
More efficient than cohort (which requires too many healthy people to follow)

Q90. Which rate is best to compare **health status of countries**?
◦ A. Crude death rate
◦ B. Age-specific death rate
◦ C. Infant mortality rate
◦ D. Proportional mortality rate

✅ **Ans:** C. Infant mortality rate
Explanation:
IMR is **highly sensitive** to changes in health, nutrition, maternal care
Used by **UNDP, WHO** in international comparisons

Q91. Which is **not a component** of Primary Health Care as per Alma-Ata declaration?
◦ A. Provision of essential drugs
◦ B. Health education
◦ C. Mental health services
◦ D. Immunization
✅ **Ans:** C. Mental health services
Explanation:
Alma-Ata (1978) listed **8 essential services** of PHC:
Health education
Food/nutrition
Safe water
Immunization
MCH
Essential drugs
Endemic disease control
Treatment of common illnesses
Mental health wasn't explicitly included.

Q92. Which is the **most appropriate measure of central tendency** for a skewed distribution?
◦ A. Mean
◦ B. Median
◦ C. Mode
◦ D. Standard deviation
✅ **Ans:** B. Median
Explanation:
Median is robust to **extreme values**
In skewed data:
Mean is dragged toward tail
Median remains central
Used in income, population studies

Q93. Which term refers to **non-random association between exposure and outcome due to a third factor**?
◦ A. Bias
◦ B. Confounding
◦ C. Effect modification
◦ D. Correlation
✅ **Ans:** B. Confounding
Explanation:
Confounding = mixing of effects
E.g., smoking → alcohol → heart disease
Smoking may confound the alcohol–heart link

Q94. A study that includes all **cases of diarrhea** admitted to hospital in a month is:
◦ A. Case series
◦ B. Case-control
◦ C. Cross-sectional
◦ D. Ecological
✅ **Ans:** A. Case series
Explanation:
Case series = descriptive study on multiple **known cases**, no comparison
Helpful in outbreak detection, early clues

Q95. Which vaccine is **not given in pregnancy**?
◦ A. TT
◦ B. Td
◦ C. MMR
◦ D. Hepatitis B
✅ **Ans:** C. MMR
Explanation:
MMR is a **live attenuated vaccine →**

contraindicated
Safe in pregnancy: TT, Td, Hep B, inactivated flu

Q96. Which of the following has **maximum influence on vaccine cold chain failure**?
◦ A. Freeze-sensitivity
◦ B. Heat sensitivity
◦ C. Vial monitor
◦ D. Adverse events

✅ **Ans:** B. Heat sensitivity
Explanation:
Live vaccines are highly heat-sensitive (e.g., OPV, BCG, measles)
Heat is the **most common cold chain failure** cause in field settings

---

Q97. What is the **numerator** in Infant Mortality Rate (IMR)?
◦ A. Infant deaths under 1 year
◦ B. Neonatal deaths
◦ C. Under-five deaths
◦ D. Perinatal deaths

✅ **Ans:** A. Infant deaths under 1 year
Explanation:
IMR = (Deaths <1 year / Live births) × 1000

Q98. What is the **critical characteristic of sentinel surveillance**?
◦ A. Reports all cases
◦ B. Detects emerging epidemics
◦ C. Conducted by every PHC
◦ D. Includes only non-communicable diseases

✅ **Ans:** B. Detects emerging epidemics
Explanation:
Sentinel = selected sites monitor **trends, alerts** → early warning
Doesn't capture every case (not exhaustive)

Q99. Which vaccine is given **at birth** as per National Immunization Schedule?
◦ A. Measles
◦ B. Pentavalent
◦ C. BCG
◦ D. DPT

✅ **Ans:** C. BCG
Explanation:
Birth vaccines:
BCG
OPV 0
Hepatitis B 0

Q100. A person returns from cholera-affected area. He is **asymptomatic but infectious**. He is:
◦ A. Primary case
◦ B. Secondary case
◦ C. Carrier
◦ D. Subclinical case

✅ **Ans:** C. Carrier
Explanation:
Carrier = person who harbors pathogen, no symptoms, can transmit
Subclinical = has internal illness but no signs (not necessarily infectious)

Q101. Which of the following is true regarding the Salk vaccine?
◦ A. Live vaccine
◦ B. Given orally
◦ C. Killed vaccine
◦ D. Provides mucosal immunity

✅ **Ans:** C. Killed vaccine
Explanation:
Salk vaccine = IPV (Inactivated Polio Vaccine)
Killed virus

Given IM
Provides **humoral immunity**
Contrast:
OPV = live, oral, mucosal + systemic immunity

Q102. A patient with COVID-19 infection but no symptoms is placed in home isolation. This is an example of:
◦ A. Isolation
◦ B. Quarantine
◦ C. Segregation
◦ D. Surveillance
✅ **Ans:** A. Isolation
Explanation:
Isolation = separating infected individuals (even asymptomatic) from healthy persons
Quarantine = separating exposed but healthy

Q103. Which is the best method to evaluate **incidence** of a disease?
◦ A. Case-control study
◦ B. Cross-sectional study
◦ C. Prospective cohort study
◦ D. Ecological study
✅ **Ans:** C. Prospective cohort study
Explanation:
Only **cohort studies** (especially prospective) can calculate **incidence**, relative risk
Others are retrospective or do not follow over time

Q104. Which statistical test is used to assess the **association between two categorical variables**?
◦ A. t-test
◦ B. ANOVA
◦ C. Chi-square test
◦ D. Z-test
✅ **Ans:** C. Chi-square test
Explanation:
Chi-square = used for **nominal data**, e.g., gender vs disease status
t-test = continuous variables, ANOVA = >2 group means

Q105. What is the vector of Japanese Encephalitis in India?
◦ A. Aedes
◦ B. Anopheles
◦ C. Culex
◦ D. Tsetse fly
✅ **Ans:** C. Culex
Explanation:
Culex vishnui complex → breeds in **rice fields**, transmits JE
Pigs = amplifier host
Ardeid birds = reservoir

Q106. An individual gets a positive Mantoux test without symptoms of TB. This is:
◦ A. Disease
◦ B. Carrier
◦ C. Subclinical infection
◦ D. Incubation
✅ **Ans:** C. Subclinical infection
Explanation:
Subclinical = infection without symptoms, but with immune response or lab markers
Carrier = asymptomatic but capable of transmission

Q107. A person develops disease after consuming contaminated water. This is an example of:
◦ A. Vehicle-borne transmission
◦ B. Vector-borne

◦ C. Airborne
◦ D. Contact

✅ **Ans:** A. Vehicle-borne transmission

Explanation:

Vehicle = **non-living medium** like water, food, blood

Vector = insects

Contact = direct person-person

Q108. Which is **not a live vaccine**?
◦ A. MMR
◦ B. BCG
◦ C. Hepatitis B
◦ D. OPV

✅ **Ans:** C. Hepatitis B

Explanation:

Hep B = **recombinant subunit vaccine**

Live vaccines include:

MMR

BCG

OPV

Yellow fever

Q109. A test that identifies almost all diseased individuals but also some healthy ones is:
◦ A. Highly specific
◦ B. Highly sensitive
◦ C. Low PPV
◦ D. Low NPV

✅ **Ans:** B. Highly sensitive

Explanation:

High sensitivity → **low false negatives**, may have **more false positives**

Useful for **screening**

Q110. Which country does **not** fall under the WHO South-East Asia Region (SEARO)?
◦ A. India
◦ B. Indonesia
◦ C. Bangladesh
◦ D. China

✅ **Ans:** D. China

Explanation:

China is in **WHO Western Pacific Region**, not SEARO

SEARO includes India, Bangladesh, Indonesia, Thailand, Nepal, etc.

Q111. Which is the **index case** in an epidemic?
◦ A. First diagnosed case
◦ B. First case in the community
◦ C. Last case in epidemic
◦ D. Most symptomatic case

✅ **Ans:** A. First diagnosed case

Explanation:

Index case = first case brought to notice of health authorities

Not always the first person to get the disease (that's the **primary case**)

Q112. Which is the **most sensitive indicator** of iodine deficiency in a population?
◦ A. Goiter rate
◦ B. Neonatal TSH
◦ C. Serum T4
◦ D. Urinary iodine excretion

✅ **Ans:** D. Urinary iodine excretion

Explanation:

Best **sensitive marker** of recent intake

<100 μg/L = deficient

Goiter = long-term marker

Q113. Which health program includes **Janani Suraksha Yojana** under it?
◦ A. RMNCH+A
◦ B. RBSK
◦ C. Ayushman Bharat
◦ D. NHM

✅ **Ans:** A. RMNCH+A
Explanation:
JSY falls under **Reproductive, Maternal, Neonatal, Child & Adolescent Health (RMNCH+A)**
Part of NRHM/NUHM umbrella

Q114. A high **positive predictive value** is associated with:
◦ A. Low specificity
◦ B. High prevalence
◦ C. Low sensitivity
◦ D. Low incidence
✅ **Ans:** B. High prevalence
Explanation:
PPV increases with higher disease prevalence
Remember:
PPV = TP / (TP + FP)
High prevalence → more TP → higher PPV

Q115. Which health program provides **free transport, diet, diagnostics** to pregnant women?
◦ A. JSY
◦ B. RBSK
◦ C. JSSK
◦ D. PMSMA
✅ **Ans:** C. Janani Shishu Suraksha Karyakram (JSSK)
Explanation:
JSSK = full **maternity entitlement**:
Free delivery
Free C-section
Free drugs, tests, diet, transport
JSY = only **cash incentive**

Q116. Which type of study is a **longitudinal observational** study?
◦ A. Case-control
◦ B. Cross-sectional
◦ C. Cohort
◦ D. Ecological
✅ **Ans:** C. Cohort
Explanation:
Cohort = **follow-up over time**
It can be prospective or retrospective
Cross-sectional = snapshot
Case-control = retrospective but no follow-up

Q117. Best method to **compare birth weights** in three groups of pregnant women?
◦ A. Chi-square
◦ B. t-test
◦ C. ANOVA
◦ D. Regression
✅ **Ans:** C. ANOVA
Explanation:
ANOVA = compare means of ≥3 groups
If just 2 groups → use t-test
Chi-square = categorical data

Q118. The natural reservoir of plague is:
◦ A. Humans
◦ B. Fleas
◦ C. Rats
◦ D. Mites
✅ **Ans:** C. Rats
Explanation:
Plague:
Reservoir = rodents (rats)
Vector = **Xenopsylla flea**

Q119. A measure of **severity** of a disease is:
◦ A. Incidence
◦ B. Case Fatality Rate

◦ C. Prevalence
◦ D. Attack rate

✅ **Ans:** B. Case Fatality Rate

Explanation:

CFR = proportion of **deaths among diagnosed cases**

Used in outbreaks to understand lethality

Q120.

A program evaluating **outcome at patient level** is assessing:

◦ A. Input
◦ B. Process
◦ C. Output
◦ D. Impact

✅ **Ans:** D. Impact

Explanation:

Input = resources
Process = activity
Output = immediate result
Impact = long-term effect (e.g., reduced mortality)

Q121. Which of the following is **NOT** included in DALY?

◦ A. Years of life lost due to premature mortality
◦ B. Years lived with disability
◦ C. Life expectancy at birth
◦ D. Disability weight

✅ **Ans:** C. Life expectancy at birth

Explanation:

DALY = YLL + YLD
YLL = years of life lost
YLD = years lived with disability
Disability weight is assigned based on severity
Life expectancy is not a DALY component.

Q122. Which of the following diseases has been **eradicated globally**?

◦ A. Polio
◦ B. Smallpox
◦ C. Guinea worm
◦ D. Leprosy

✅ **Ans:** B. Smallpox

Explanation:

Smallpox eradicated in 1980 (last case 1977 Somalia)
Polio not yet eradicated globally
Guinea worm nearing eradication
Leprosy is **eliminated** from India but not eradicated

Q123. Which of the following is most reliable for **nutritional assessment** of a community?

◦ A. BMI
◦ B. Weight-for-height
◦ C. Mid-upper arm circumference
◦ D. Weight-for-age

✅ **Ans:** B. Weight-for-height

Explanation:

Weight-for-height = best indicator of **acute malnutrition**
Weight-for-age = influenced by both acute + chronic
MUAC = screening tool
BMI = general adult measure

Q124. Which vitamin deficiency is screened using **Bitot's spots**?

◦ A. A
◦ B. B1
◦ C. C
◦ D. D

✅ **Ans:** A. Vitamin A

Explanation:

Bitot's spots = triangular foamy patches on conjunctiva → sign of

Vitamin A deficiency
Also causes xerophthalmia, night blindness, keratomalacia

Q125. Most common **cause of maternal mortality** in India:
◦ A. Hemorrhage
◦ B. Sepsis
◦ C. Obstructed labor
◦ D. Eclampsia
✅ **Ans:** A. Hemorrhage
Explanation:
PPH (Postpartum Hemorrhage) is the leading cause in India & worldwide
Followed by hypertensive disorders, sepsis, unsafe abortion

Q126. Under Ayushman Bharat, the **primary health infrastructure is renamed as**:
◦ A. PHC
◦ B. Wellness center
◦ C. Subcenter
◦ D. Swasthya Mitra
✅ **Ans:** B. Wellness center
Explanation:
Ayushman Bharat has 2 components:
Health & Wellness Centers (HWCs) – upgraded SCs & PHCs
PM-JAY – insurance coverage

Q127. Which of the following is a **component of primordial prevention**?
◦ A. Vaccination
◦ B. Reducing salt in food industry
◦ C. Screening
◦ D. Physiotherapy
✅ **Ans:** B. Reducing salt in food industry
Explanation:
Primordial = preventing risk factor development itself
E.g., policies, food laws, lifestyle education

Q128. A pregnant woman with anemia (Hb 9.5 g%) comes for antenatal checkup. What is the classification?
◦ A. Mild anemia
◦ B. Moderate anemia
◦ C. Severe anemia
◦ D. Very severe
✅ **Ans:** B. Moderate anemia
Explanation (WHO classification in pregnancy):
Mild = 10–10.9
Moderate = 7–9.9
Severe = <7 g/dL

Q129. Which is **not a direct transmission** route?
◦ A. Droplet infection
◦ B. Skin contact
◦ C. Fomite
◦ D. Transplacental
✅ **Ans:** C. Fomite
Explanation:
Fomite = **indirect transmission** via inanimate objects
Direct: touch, droplet, sexual, transplacental

Q130. Which disease is **under elimination** as per India's NTD targets?
◦ A. Measles
◦ B. Malaria
◦ C. Lymphatic filariasis
◦ D. Polio
✅ **Ans:** C. Lymphatic filariasis
Explanation:
Target = eliminate LF by **2030**
Polio = eradicated from India

Malaria → elimination planned
Measles = elimination goal by 2023–25

Q131. A woman is screened for breast cancer using mammography. She has no complaints. This is an example of:
◦ A. Primordial prevention
◦ B. Primary prevention
◦ C. Secondary prevention
◦ D. Tertiary prevention
✅ **Ans:** C. Secondary prevention
Explanation:
Secondary = early detection in asymptomatic individuals, to reduce complications
e.g., mammography, Pap smear, HIV testing

Q132. Which condition is **notifiable** under IDSP in India?
◦ A. Diabetes
◦ B. Hypertension
◦ C. Dengue
◦ D. Cancer
✅ **Ans:** C. Dengue
Explanation:
IDSP (Integrated Disease Surveillance Program) covers **epidemic-prone diseases** like dengue, malaria, JE, cholera
Non-communicables like DM, HTN not included in IDSP

Q133. An outbreak with **multiple peaks** spaced by incubation periods is likely due to:
◦ A. Point source
◦ B. Continuous exposure
◦ C. Propagated outbreak
◦ D. Random spread
✅ **Ans:** C. Propagated outbreak
Explanation:
Propagated = person-to-person → multiple waves
e.g., measles, flu
Each peak = new generation of spread

Q134. Which level of prevention is **screening for hypertension** in healthy adults?
◦ A. Primordial
◦ B. Primary
◦ C. Secondary
◦ D. Tertiary
✅ **Ans:** C. Secondary
Explanation:
Detecting disease **before symptoms** = secondary
Blood pressure checks, blood sugar tests = classic examples

Q135. Which vaccine is stored in **ice-lined refrigerator (ILR)** at 2–8°C?
◦ A. OPV
◦ B. BCG
◦ C. DPT
◦ D. Measles
✅ **Ans:** C. DPT
Explanation:
DPT is freeze-sensitive, stored in ILR at **2–8°C**
ILR = deep, chest-style fridge used in UIP
OPV, BCG, Measles → stored in freezer

Q136. Which statistical test compares **proportions** of male vs female smokers in a class?
◦ A. t-test
◦ B. Chi-square
◦ C. ANOVA
◦ D. Z-test

✅ **Ans:** B. Chi-square
Explanation:
Chi-square = compares **categorical variables**
Male/female = nominal
Smoker/non-smoker = categorical

Q137. Prevalence increases, but **incidence remains constant**. What could be the reason?
◦ A. Reduced diagnosis
◦ B. Shorter duration
◦ C. Increased cure rate
◦ D. Prolonged survival
✅ **Ans:** D. Prolonged survival
Explanation:
Prevalence = Incidence × Duration
If survival improves → longer duration → prevalence increases

---

Q138. A **health assistant** is posted at which level of healthcare?
◦ A. Subcenter
◦ B. PHC
◦ C. CHC
◦ D. District hospital
✅ **Ans:** A. Subcenter
Explanation:
Subcenter staff includes:
1 ANM + 1 Male Health Worker
1 Health Assistant (female or male)

Q139. A bar diagram is best used to show:
◦ A. Frequency of categories
◦ B. Correlation
◦ C. Normal distribution
◦ D. Cumulative trend
✅ **Ans:** A. Frequency of categories
Explanation:
Bar chart = displays discrete variables (e.g., gender, literacy)
Height = frequency

Q140. Which of the following is a **biological transmission**?
◦ A. Plague by flea
◦ B. Cholera by water
◦ C. Typhoid by food
◦ D. Conjunctivitis by fingers
✅ **Ans:** A. Plague by flea
Explanation:
Biological transmission = pathogen multiplies/develops inside vector
Flea → Yersinia pestis matures inside → transmitted via bite
Others = mechanical or vehicle

Q141. Which of the following is **not a feature of a good screening test**?
◦ A. High sensitivity
◦ B. Low cost
◦ C. High specificity
◦ D. Low prevalence of disease
✅ **Ans:** D. Low prevalence of disease
Explanation:
A good screening test should be applied to **conditions with high prevalence**, so PPV is acceptable.
Low prevalence = ↓ PPV → more false positives

Q142. Which measure is used to assess **chronic undernutrition** in children?
◦ A. Weight-for-age
◦ B. MUAC
◦ C. Height-for-age
◦ D. Weight-for-height
✅ **Ans:** C. Height-for-age
Explanation:
Height-for-age = **stunting**, indicates long-standing malnutrition

Weight-for-height = acute
MUAC = field screening

Q143. Which statistical test is used for association between **education level and tobacco use**?
◦ A. t-test
◦ B. ANOVA
◦ C. Chi-square test
◦ D. Pearson correlation

✅ **Ans:** C. Chi-square test
Explanation:
Both education and tobacco use are **categorical variables**
Chi-square = best for checking association between **two qualitative variables**

Q144. Which mosquito can transmit **more than one disease**?
◦ A. Anopheles
◦ B. Culex
◦ C. Aedes
◦ D. Mansonia

✅ **Ans:** C. Aedes
Explanation:
Aedes aegypti transmits:
Dengue
Chikungunya
Zika
Yellow fever
Also day-biting & breeds in clean water

Q145. A woman delivers at home with help of a trained dai. What is this level of care?
◦ A. Primary
◦ B. Secondary
◦ C. Tertiary
◦ D. Community-based

✅ **Ans:** A. Primary
Explanation:
Home-based care by **trained birth attendants** is part of **primary care**
Referral to PHC/CHC if complications arise

Q146. Which of the following increases the **specificity** of a screening program?
◦ A. Repeat test
◦ B. Use of sensitive test
◦ C. Use of confirmatory test
◦ D. Use of low cutoff

✅ **Ans:** C. Use of confirmatory test
Explanation:
Screening = high sensitivity
Confirmation = high specificity
Confirmatory tests reduce **false positives**

Q147. A vaccine vial monitor turns dark. What does it mean?
◦ A. Frozen
◦ B. Vaccine safe
◦ C. Heat exposed & ineffective
◦ D. Cold chain intact

✅ **Ans:** C. Heat exposed & ineffective
Explanation:
VVM darkens irreversibly if exposed to heat → vaccine should be discarded
Particularly used with OPV

Q148. What is the **normal range of BMI** as per WHO for adults?
◦ A. 18.5–24.9
◦ B. 20–25
◦ C. 18–26
◦ D. 17–22

✅ **Ans:** A. 18.5–24.9
Explanation:
<18.5 = underweight
18.5–24.9 = normal

25–29.9 = overweight
≥30 = obese

Q149. Which committee recommended **three-tier health system** in India?
◦ A. Bhore
◦ B. Mudaliar
◦ C. Shrivastav
◦ D. Kartar Singh
✅ **Ans:** A. Bhore Committee (1946)
Explanation:
Bhore Committee → foundation of Indian PHC system
Subcenter → PHC → CHC
Also proposed **integration of preventive & curative services**

Q150. Which type of bias is seen if interviewer probes cases more than controls?
◦ A. Recall bias
◦ B. Selection bias
◦ C. Interviewer bias
◦ D. Confounding
✅ **Ans:** C. Interviewer bias
Explanation:
Interviewer bias = unequal questioning between groups
Can be minimized via **blinding, structured questionnaire**

Q151. Which health committee introduced the concept of **"health worker for every village"**?
◦ A. Bhore Committee
◦ B. Shrivastav Committee
◦ C. Mudaliar Committee
◦ D. Jungalwalla Committee
✅ **Ans:** B. Shrivastav Committee
Explanation:
1975 – **Shrivastav Committee** recommended:
Community-based workers (like ASHA)
Creation of a **cadre of health volunteers**

Q152. A **cohort study** has been conducted. Which value can it directly measure?
◦ A. Odds ratio
◦ B. Prevalence
◦ C. Attributable risk
◦ D. Sensitivity
✅ **Ans:** C. Attributable risk
Explanation:
Cohort studies allow:
Incidence
Relative risk
Attributable risk
(OR is from case-control; sensitivity is from diagnostics)

Q153. What is the **incubation period of dengue**?
◦ A. 1–3 days
◦ B. 4–7 days
◦ C. 10–14 days
◦ D. 14–21 days
✅ **Ans:** B. 4–7 days
Explanation:
Dengue fever:
Incubation = 4–7 days (range 3–10)
Virus: Flavivirus (Aedes vector)

Q154. Which is **not** a mode of intervention in primary prevention?
◦ A. Health education
◦ B. Chemoprophylaxis
◦ C. Early diagnosis
◦ D. Vaccination

✅ **Ans:** C. Early diagnosis

Explanation:

Early diagnosis = **secondary prevention**

Primary prevention = health promotion (education) + specific protection (vaccines, chemoprophylaxis)

Q155. Which test gives **maximum information about a diagnostic test's utility in ruling out disease**?

- A. Sensitivity
- B. Specificity
- C. Negative predictive value
- D. Positive predictive value

✅ **Ans:** C. Negative predictive value

Explanation:

NPV = probability that a person with negative result is truly disease-free

High NPV = **good for ruling out**

Q156. A study involving 1000 people assesses their height and hemoglobin on the same day. Type of study?

- A. Cohort
- B. Cross-sectional
- C. Case-control
- D. Experimental

✅ **Ans:** B. Cross-sectional

Explanation:

Cross-sectional = **snapshot in time**

Good for measuring **prevalence**, associations (not cause-effect)

Q157. A patient bitten by a dog receives ARV + RIG. What type of immunization is this?

- A. Active
- B. Passive
- C. Both
- D. None

✅ **Ans:** C. Both

Explanation:

ARV (vaccine) = **active**

RIG (immunoglobulin) = **passive**

Given together in **Category III exposures**

Q158. Which vaccine is **most heat-sensitive**?

- A. BCG
- B. DPT
- C. OPV
- D. Hep B

✅ **Ans:** C. OPV

Explanation:

OPV (Sabin vaccine) is **most heat-sensitive** in UIP

Requires cold chain; potency drops fast if exposed to heat

Q159. A patient tests positive in a **low prevalence setting**. What will happen to PPV?

- A. Increases
- B. Decreases
- C. No change
- D. Variable

✅ **Ans:** B. Decreases

Explanation:

PPV ↓ when prevalence ↓

Because false positives rise in low-prevalence settings

Q160. What does a **right-skewed curve** indicate?

- A. Mean > Median > Mode
- B. Median > Mean > Mode
- C. Mode > Mean > Median
- D. Mean = Median = Mode

✅ **Ans:** A. Mean > Median > Mode

Explanation:

Right skew (positive skew) = long tail to right
Mean pulled higher than median or mode

Q161. Which program provides **weekly iron-folic acid supplementation** to adolescents?
◦ A. RBSK
◦ B. WIFS
◦ C. JSY
◦ D. JSSK
✅ **Ans:** B. WIFS (Weekly Iron and Folic acid Supplementation)
Explanation:
Targets **10–19-year-olds**
IFA tablet weekly (blue for adolescents)
Deworming bi-annually

Q162. What is the **population covered** by a PHC in a plain area in India?
◦ A. 10,000
◦ B. 20,000
◦ C. 30,000
◦ D. 50,000
✅ **Ans:** C. 30,000
Explanation:
PHC coverage:
Plains = 30,000
Hilly/tribal = 20,000
CHC: 1 per 1.2 lakh (plain)

Q163. Which of the following is an **active artificial immunity**?
◦ A. Antitoxin administration
◦ B. Immunoglobulin therapy
◦ C. Natural infection
◦ D. Vaccination
✅ **Ans:** D. Vaccination
Explanation:
Active = body produces antibody
→ Natural (infection), Artificial (vaccination)
Passive = ready-made antibody (Ig, antitoxin)

Q164. Which vitamin is given in management of **measles** in children?
◦ A. Vitamin A
◦ B. Vitamin B12
◦ C. Vitamin D
◦ D. Vitamin C
✅ **Ans:** A. Vitamin A
Explanation:
WHO recommends 2 doses of Vitamin A for all children with measles
→ reduces complications, mortality

Q165. Which of the following is **not a water-borne disease**?
◦ A. Hepatitis A
◦ B. Cholera
◦ C. Typhoid
◦ D. Dengue
✅ **Ans:** D. Dengue
Explanation:
Dengue = **Aedes mosquito-borne**
Others → water/food contamination

Q166. Which organization **certifies countries polio-free**?
◦ A. UNICEF
◦ B. ICMR
◦ C. WHO
◦ D. NITI Aayog
✅ **Ans:** C. WHO
Explanation:
WHO certifies polio-free status after 3 years of zero wild virus transmission
India certified polio-free in 2014

Q167. Which vaccine requires **diluent** during administration?
◦ A. OPV
◦ B. DPT
◦ C. BCG
◦ D. Hepatitis B

✅ **Ans:** C. BCG

Explanation:
BCG & Measles vaccines come as **lyophilized powder** → reconstituted with sterile diluent

---

Q168. Which mosquito has **nocturnal feeding** and breeds in **polluted water**?
◦ A. Aedes
◦ B. Culex
◦ C. Anopheles
◦ D. Mansonia

✅ **Ans:** B. Culex

Explanation:
Culex → night biter
Breeds in **stagnant polluted water** (gutters, septic tanks)
Vector for JE, filariasis

Q169. Which mosquito has **short flight range** and **multiple feeding habits**?
◦ A. Aedes
◦ B. Culex
◦ C. Anopheles
◦ D. Mansonia

✅ **Ans:** A. Aedes

Explanation:
Aedes aegypti:
Flight range <100 m
Day biter
Prefers human blood (anthropophilic)
Multiple bites = ↑ transmission

Q170. In cohort studies, outcome can be affected by **loss to follow-up**, leading to:
◦ A. Measurement bias
◦ B. Observer bias
◦ C. Selection bias
◦ D. Confounding

✅ **Ans:** C. Selection bias

Explanation:
When **exposed and unexposed groups** lose participants unequally → skewed results
Selection bias = **differential attrition**

Q171. Which part of ice-lined refrigerator (ILR) should **vaccine vials never touch**?
◦ A. Sides
◦ B. Bottom
◦ C. Middle
◦ D. Top

✅ **Ans:** B. Bottom

Explanation:
In ILRs, direct contact with bottom may cause **freezing** of vaccines
Vaccines should be kept **in baskets**, away from bottom and sides

---

Q172. Which of the following is **not used for herd immunity calculation**?
◦ A. R_0
◦ B. Vaccine efficacy
◦ C. Duration of immunity
◦ D. Relative risk

✅ **Ans:** D. Relative risk

Explanation:
Herd immunity threshold = $1 - (1/R_0)$
Depends on infectivity (R_0), immunity duration, vaccine coverage
Relative risk is **study output**, not immunity factor

Q173. Which of the following best defines **reproductive rate (R_0)**?
◦ A. Average no. of deaths per 1000
◦ B. Avg. no. of births per couple
◦ C. Avg. no. of secondary cases from one case
◦ D. Lifetime fertility

✅ **Ans:** C. Avg. no. of secondary cases from one case

Explanation:
R_0 = **transmission potential** of a disease in a completely susceptible population
Measles R_0 ~15–18, COVID ~2–3

Q174. Which disease is transmitted via **cyclopropagative transmission**?
◦ A. Malaria
◦ B. Yellow fever
◦ C. Dengue
◦ D. Leptospirosis

✅ **Ans:** A. Malaria

Explanation:
Cyclopropagative = multiplication + development in vector
Malaria (Plasmodium in Anopheles)
Cyclodevelopmental = Filaria
Propagative = plague, dengue

Q175. Which of the following is **not part of cold chain**?
◦ A. Vaccine carrier
◦ B. Deep freezer
◦ C. Cold box
◦ D. Needle hub

✅ **Ans:** D. Needle hub

Explanation:
Cold chain = equipment used to **store, transport vaccines** at correct temperatures
Needles/syringes are not part of cold chain.

Q176. Which schedule vaccine is **not given through UIP** in private clinics?
◦ A. OPV
◦ B. Pentavalent
◦ C. PCV
◦ D. Rotavirus

✅ **Ans:** C. PCV

Explanation:
Pneumococcal Conjugate Vaccine (PCV) is given in selected states via UIP
Private sector may provide it, but not universally
(Answer may vary based on year/state rollouts)

Q177. Which disease has **airborne transmission**?
◦ A. Hepatitis A
◦ B. Cholera
◦ C. Tuberculosis
◦ D. Typhoid

✅ **Ans:** C. Tuberculosis

Explanation:
TB = classic **airborne infection**
Droplet nuclei remain suspended → highly infectious
Others = fecal-oral

Q178. Ideal epidemiological unit for surveillance?
◦ A. Village
◦ B. PHC
◦ C. Subcenter
◦ D. Household

✅ **Ans:** B. PHC

Explanation:
PHC = central unit for health data

reporting, surveillance, interventions
Each PHC covers ~30,000 in plains

Q179. Which of the following is used in **national nutritional anemia prophylaxis**?

◦ A. Iron alone
◦ B. Iron + folic acid
◦ C. Iron + vitamin A
◦ D. Iron + zinc

✅ **Ans:** B. Iron + folic acid

Explanation:
All age groups get **iron + folic acid** in varying dosages and frequencies
e.g., pink tablet for 5–9 yrs, red for pregnant women

Q180. Which of the following reflects **true vaccine efficacy in community**?

◦ A. Efficacy
◦ B. Effectiveness
◦ C. Efficiency
◦ D. Immunogenicity

✅ **Ans:** B. Effectiveness

Explanation:
Effectiveness = performance in **real-world conditions**
Efficacy = ideal conditions (e.g., clinical trials)

Q181. A 6-month-old infant is brought for DPT3. He has mild fever. What is the next step?

◦ A. Defer vaccine
◦ B. Give DPT3
◦ C. Give DPT after antibiotics
◦ D. Give only DT

✅ **Ans:** B. Give DPT3

Explanation:
Mild fever, cough, cold are not contraindications
Only moderate/severe illness, convulsions, or hypersensitivity are reasons to defer

---

Q182. Which of the following diseases is **notifiable** in India?

◦ A. Hypertension
◦ B. Diabetes
◦ C. HIV/AIDS
◦ D. Asthma

✅ **Ans:** C. HIV/AIDS

Explanation:
Since 2012, **HIV/AIDS** is notifiable
→ Helps planning ART services
Others are NCDs, not under notifiable list

Q183. Which indicator is used to monitor the **magnitude of an epidemic**?

◦ A. Incidence rate
◦ B. Prevalence
◦ C. Secondary attack rate
◦ D. Case fatality rate

✅ **Ans:** A. Incidence rate

Explanation:
Incidence = new cases
Tracks how fast disease is spreading
CFR = severity; SAR = spread among contacts

Q184. Which is the most appropriate **visual display** for comparing literacy rates of different states?

◦ A. Line graph
◦ B. Bar chart
◦ C. Pie chart
◦ D. Histogram

✅ **Ans:** B. Bar chart

Explanation:
Bar = best for **categorical/discrete variables** like state-wise literacy

Line = trends over time
Pie = parts of a whole

Q185. An outbreak of hepatitis A occurs in a school. Best control measure?
◦ A. Isolation
◦ B. Passive immunization
◦ C. Water sanitation
◦ D. Antibiotics
✅ **Ans:** C. Water sanitation
Explanation:
Hep A = **fecal-oral** → spread due to contaminated food/water
Prevented by hygiene, safe water, hygiene education

Q186. Which vaccine should be **discarded 4 hours** after reconstitution?
◦ A. BCG
◦ B. Measles
◦ C. TT
◦ D. Hepatitis B
✅ **Ans:** A. BCG
Explanation:
Reconstituted BCG must be used within **4–6 hours**
Measles → up to 6 hours
Others (liquid form) follow VVM & expiry

Q187. Which statistical value remains **unaffected by outliers**?
◦ A. Mean
◦ B. Standard deviation
◦ C. Range
◦ D. Median
✅ **Ans:** D. Median
Explanation:
Median = middle value
Robust to extreme values
Mean & SD get pulled by outliers

Q188. Which of the following represents **secondary prevention** in cancer?
◦ A. Chemotherapy
◦ B. Palliative care
◦ C. Pap smear
◦ D. Health education
✅ **Ans:** C. Pap smear
Explanation:
Secondary = early detection
Pap smear, mammography, colonoscopy = screening tools

Q189. A patient is found to be infected with HIV. What is the next best public health response?
◦ A. Report to IDSP
◦ B. Start antiretroviral therapy
◦ C. Trace and counsel contacts
◦ D. Begin isolation
✅ **Ans:** C. Trace and counsel contacts
Explanation:
Contact tracing + counseling is key for preventing further transmission
ART is part of clinical care; isolation not required

Q190. A false positive result increases when:
◦ A. Specificity decreases
◦ B. Sensitivity decreases
◦ C. Prevalence increases
◦ D. PPV increases
✅ **Ans:** A. Specificity decreases
Explanation:
Low specificity = more false positives
Important in confirmatory testing

Q191.
Which is the **most important component** of RCH (Reproductive and Child Health)?
◦ A. Family planning
◦ B. Adolescent health
◦ C. Skilled birth attendance
◦ D. Immunization
✅ **Ans:** C. Skilled birth attendance
Explanation:
SBA directly reduces maternal/neonatal deaths
Core of safe motherhood strategy

Q192. What does the **yellow color bag** in BMW management carry?
◦ A. Soiled linen
◦ B. Used IV sets
◦ C. Syringes
◦ D. Ampoules
✅ **Ans:** A. Soiled linen
Explanation:
BMW 2016 rules:
Yellow = human waste, soiled items
Red = plastics
White = sharps
Blue = glass

Q193. A case-control study gives us:
◦ A. Relative risk
◦ B. Attributable risk
◦ C. Odds ratio
◦ D. Prevalence
✅ **Ans:** C. Odds ratio
Explanation:
Case-control → Odds ratio
Can't get incidence or RR because you start with cases

Q194. Which of the following **reduces prevalence** of a disease?
◦ A. Early diagnosis
◦ B. Reduced incidence
◦ C. Improved survival
◦ D. Migration of cases
✅ **Ans:** B. Reduced incidence
Explanation:
Prevalence = incidence × duration
So reducing **new cases** lowers prevalence

Q195. Which term refers to **detecting disease before symptoms appear**?
◦ A. Primary prevention
◦ B. Secondary prevention
◦ C. Tertiary prevention
◦ D. Quaternary prevention
✅ **Ans:** B. Secondary prevention
Explanation:
Screening = hallmark of secondary prevention
(e.g., Pap smear, BP check)

Q196. Highest **case fatality rate** is seen in:
◦ A. Influenza
◦ B. Ebola
◦ C. Measles
◦ D. Tuberculosis
✅ **Ans:** B. Ebola
Explanation:
Ebola has CFR > 50–80%
Used to indicate **lethality** in infected population

Q197. Most common mode of **HIV transmission in India**?
◦ A. Blood transfusion
◦ B. Heterosexual contact
◦ C. Vertical
◦ D. IVDU

✅ **Ans:** B. Heterosexual contact

Explanation:

85% of cases in India via heterosexual route

High-risk behaviors → key target for prevention

Q198. Line listing is used in:

◦ A. Outbreak investigation

◦ B. Immunization program

◦ C. Birth registration

◦ D. Census

✅ **Ans:** A. Outbreak investigation

Explanation:

Line list = **tabular form of individual case details**

Helps cluster analysis, contact tracing

Q199. Ice packs in vaccine carriers should be conditioned before use to:

◦ A. Prevent heat exposure

◦ B. Prevent freezing vaccines

◦ C. Maintain sterility

◦ D. Reduce weight

✅ **Ans:** B. Prevent freezing vaccines

Explanation:

Conditioning = partially melting ice packs

→ prevents freeze-sensitive vaccines (DPT, TT) from damage

Q200. A health policy bans smoking in public places. This is an example of:

◦ A. Primordial prevention

◦ B. Primary prevention

◦ C. Secondary prevention

◦ D. Tertiary prevention

✅ **Ans:** A. Primordial prevention

Explanation:

Primordial = prevent emergence of risk factors (e.g., tobacco use)

Policy level intervention

Bonus PSM Revision

Q1. Which mosquito causes daytime bite and spreads dengue?
◦ A. Anopheles
◦ B. Aedes
◦ C. Culex
◦ D. Mansonia
✓ **Ans:** B. Aedes

Q2. Which index is most sensitive for community health status?
◦ A. Crude death rate
◦ B. IMR
◦ C. Life expectancy
◦ D. Birth rate
✓ **Ans:** B. IMR

Q3. Which vaccine is most heat-sensitive in UIP?
◦ A. DPT
◦ B. Hepatitis B
◦ C. OPV
◦ D. TT
✓ **Ans:** C. OPV

Q4. BCG is administered via:
◦ A. Intradermal
◦ B. Subcutaneous
◦ C. IM
◦ D. Oral
✓ **Ans:** A. Intradermal

Q5. Target year for TB elimination in India:
◦ A. 2022
◦ B. 2023
◦ C. 2025
◦ D. 2030
✓ **Ans:** C. 2025

Q6. Which is not a component of ASHA's role?
◦ A. Conducting deliveries
◦ B. Mobilizing community
◦ C. Health education
◦ D. Linking to health services
✓ **Ans:** A. Conducting deliveries

Q7. Universal Immunization Program was launched in:
◦ A. 1983
◦ B. 1985
◦ C. 1986
◦ D. 1992
✓ **Ans:** B. 1985

Q8. What is the denominator for MMR?
◦ A. Total pregnancies
◦ B. Total births
◦ C. Live births
◦ D. Stillbirths
✓ **Ans:** C. Live births

Q9. Which vitamin is supplemented under NACP (HIV program)?
◦ A. Vitamin A
◦ B. Vitamin C
◦ C. Multivitamins
◦ D. Folic acid
✓ **Ans:** C. Multivitamins

Q10. What is the method used to compare **three means**?

◦ A. t-test
◦ B. Chi-square
◦ C. ANOVA
◦ D. Correlation
✓ **Ans:** C. ANOVA

Q11. R_0 of a disease indicates:
◦ A. Case fatality rate
◦ B. Incubation period
◦ C. Secondary cases from one case
◦ D. Duration of illness
✓ **Ans:** C. Secondary cases from one case

Q12. Vector for Japanese Encephalitis in India:
◦ A. Aedes
◦ B. Culex
◦ C. Anopheles
◦ D. Mansonia
✓ **Ans:** B. Culex

Q13. DOTS strategy is used for:
◦ A. HIV
◦ B. TB
◦ C. Malaria
◦ D. Dengue
✓ **Ans:** B. TB

Q14. Which is a **late indicator** of iron deficiency?
◦ A. Serum ferritin
◦ B. Hemoglobin
◦ C. Transferrin saturation
◦ D. Serum iron
✓ **Ans:** B. Hemoglobin

Q15. Basic statistical measure for **skewed data**:
◦ A. Mean
◦ B. Mode
◦ C. Median
◦ D. Range
✓ **Ans:** C. Median

Q16. Which of the following is **freeze-sensitive**?
◦ A. OPV
◦ B. DPT
◦ C. Measles
◦ D. BCG
✓ **Ans:** B. DPT

Q17. Malaria surveillance unit at district level:
◦ A. PHC
◦ B. CHC
◦ C. DMO office
◦ D. District Malaria Office
✓ **Ans:** D. District Malaria Office

Q18. Which disease is **notifiable** under IDSP?
◦ A. Diabetes
◦ B. Dengue
◦ C. Asthma
◦ D. Hypertension
✓ **Ans:** B. Dengue

Q19. Prevalence is increased by:
◦ A. Increased mortality
◦ B. Shorter disease duration
◦ C. Chronic nature of disease
◦ D. Rapid cure
✓ **Ans:** C. Chronic nature of disease

Q20. A disease with **high infectivity, low pathogenicity** is:
◦ A. Rabies
◦ B. Influenza
◦ C. Tetanus

◦ D. Tuberculosis

✅ **Ans:** B. Influenza

Q21. Best method to measure malaria incidence in a community:

◦ A. Slide positivity rate
◦ B. Annual blood examination rate
◦ C. Annual parasite incidence
◦ D. Case fatality rate

✅ **Ans:** C. Annual parasite incidence (API)

Q22. Which mosquito lays eggs singly and has lateral floats?

◦ A. Aedes
◦ B. Anopheles
◦ C. Culex
◦ D. Mansonia

✅ **Ans:** B. Anopheles

Q23. Herd immunity **does not protect against**:

◦ A. Measles
◦ B. Rubella
◦ C. Tetanus
◦ D. Polio

✅ **Ans:** C. Tetanus

Q24. The vaccine that is **stored in deep freezer** is:

◦ A. OPV
◦ B. DPT
◦ C. Hepatitis B
◦ D. TT

✅ **Ans:** A. OPV

Q25. Live vaccines include all except:

◦ A. OPV
◦ B. MMR
◦ C. BCG
◦ D. Hepatitis B

✅ **Ans:** D. Hepatitis B

Q26. Maximum effect of health education is at:

◦ A. Knowledge level
◦ B. Attitude level
◦ C. Behavior level
◦ D. Practice level

✅ **Ans:** D. Practice level

Q27. Surveillance involving **zero reporting** is:

◦ A. Active
◦ B. Passive
◦ C. Sentinel
◦ D. Universal

✅ **Ans:** D. Universal

Q28. Most important determinant of sample size in study:

◦ A. Confidence interval
◦ B. Prevalence
◦ C. p-value
◦ D. Median

✅ **Ans:** B. Prevalence

Q29. Case detection and treatment is part of which prevention level?

◦ A. Primordial
◦ B. Primary
◦ C. Secondary
◦ D. Tertiary

✅ **Ans:** C. Secondary

Q30. The best index for assessing **obesity in adults** is:

◦ A. BMI
◦ B. Waist–hip ratio
◦ C. Skinfold thickness

◦ D. Broca's index

✅ **Ans:** A. BMI

Q41. In which phase is safety of a drug tested in healthy volunteers?

◦ A. Phase I
◦ B. Phase II
◦ C. Phase III
◦ D. Phase IV

✅ **Ans:** A. Phase I

Q42. Highest priority group for iron supplementation under Anemia Mukt Bharat?

◦ A. Pregnant women
◦ B. Postmenopausal women
◦ C. Children <5 years
◦ D. Men

✅ **Ans:** A. Pregnant women

Q43. In case-control study, **bias in recalling past exposure** is called:

◦ A. Recall bias
◦ B. Selection bias
◦ C. Observer bias
◦ D. Referral bias

✅ **Ans:** A. Recall bias

Q44. Which is a **non-communicable disease surveillance system** in India?

◦ A. IDSP
◦ B. NFHS
◦ C. DLHS
◦ D. STEPS

✅ **Ans:** D. STEPS (by WHO for NCDs)

Q45. Which organization manages **vaccine procurement and distribution** in UIP?

◦ A. WHO
◦ B. UNICEF
◦ C. Central Medical Services Society (CMSS)
◦ D. NACO

✅ **Ans:** C. CMSS

Q46. Which program provides screening for 4Ds in children?

◦ A. RBSK
◦ B. RKSK
◦ C. PMSMA
◦ D. JSSK

✅ **Ans:** A. RBSK

4Ds = Defects, Diseases, Deficiencies, Developmental delays

Q47. What is the **sampling unit** in cluster sampling?

◦ A. Individual
◦ B. Village
◦ C. Household
◦ D. Cluster

✅ **Ans:** D. Cluster

Q48. Most common **chronic occupational disease** in India:

◦ A. Silicosis
◦ B. Byssinosis
◦ C. Asbestosis
◦ D. Farmer's lung

✅ **Ans:** A. Silicosis

Q49. Under biomedical waste rules, yellow bag waste is:

◦ A. Incinerated
◦ B. Autoclaved
◦ C. Shredded
◦ D. Deep buried

✅ **Ans:** A. Incinerated

Q50. Which one of the following **statistical values** is most affected by outliers?
◦ A. Median
◦ B. Mean
◦ C. Mode
◦ D. Z-score
✓ **Ans:** B. Mean

Q51. Z-score in statistics is used to:
◦ A. Compare two means
◦ B. Measure correlation
◦ C. Standardize data
◦ D. Test significance
✓ **Ans:** C. Standardize data

Q52. Under POSHAN Abhiyan, which group is most targeted?
◦ A. Adolescents
◦ B. Pregnant and lactating women
◦ C. Elderly
D. Children with disability
Ans: B. Pregnant and lactating ıen

'Jnder NACO, which test is used 'ine screening for HIV?
ərn blot

'st

ıd test

ıminated from a ıts globally is said to

◦ D. Extinct
✓ **Ans:** B. Eliminated

Q55. Non-living agents like vehicles, water, and fomites transmit disease via:
◦ A. Contact
◦ B. Vehicle-borne transmission
◦ C. Vector
◦ D. Droplet
✓ **Ans:** B. Vehicle-borne transmission

Q56. Sentinel surveillance is best suited for:
◦ A. Complete coverage
◦ B. Trend analysis
◦ C. Eradication
◦ D. Individual diagnosis
✓ **Ans:** B. Trend analysis

Q57. Rehabilitation of a stroke patient is what level of prevention?
◦ A. Primary
◦ B. Secondary
◦ C. Tertiary
◦ D. Primordial
✓ **Ans:** C. Tertiary

Q58. If a test gives same results on repeated runs, it has:
◦ A. High validity
◦ B. High reliability
◦ C. High specificity
◦ D. High accuracy
✓ **Ans:** B. High reliability

Q59. Incubation period of **cholera** is:
◦ A. Few hours to 5 days
◦ B. 7–10 days
◦ C. 14–21 days

◦ D. 3–6 weeks

✓ **Ans:** A. Few hours to 5 days

Q60. An outbreak due to exposure to contaminated ice cream is:

◦ A. Propagated
◦ B. Point source
◦ C. Continuous exposure
◦ D. Sporadic

✓ **Ans:** B. Point source

Q61. Which vaccine is given **only in the left deltoid** in newborns?

◦ A. OPV
◦ B. BCG
◦ C. Hepatitis B
◦ D. Measles

✓ **Ans:** B. BCG

Q62. The color of bag for disposal of **IV sets and catheters** is:

◦ A. Red
◦ B. Yellow
◦ C. Blue
◦ D. White

✓ **Ans:** A. Red

Q63. Which mosquito's larvae attach to **aquatic plants**?

◦ A. Aedes
◦ B. Mansonia
◦ C. Culex
◦ D. Anopheles

✓ **Ans:** B. Mansonia

Q64. A person harbors pathogen but has **no symptoms** and **can transmit** the disease. He is a:

◦ A. Subclinical case
◦ B. Latent case
◦ C. Carrier
◦ D. Convalescent

✓ **Ans:** C. Carrier

Q65. Best sampling method for vaccinating 100 children in 10 villages:

◦ A. Simple random
◦ B. Stratified
◦ C. Systematic
◦ D. Cluster

✓ **Ans:** D. Cluster

Q66. Most specific test for surveillance of neonatal hypothyroidism:

◦ A. TSH
◦ B. T3
◦ C. T4
◦ D. Thyroglobulin

✓ **Ans:** A. TSH

Q67. Disease with **highest R_0**:

◦ A. COVID-19
◦ B. Ebola
◦ C. Measles
◦ D. Polio

✓ **Ans:** C. Measles

Q68. Which mosquito **bites multiple times** in a single meal?

◦ A. Anopheles
◦ B. Aedes
◦ C. Culex
◦ D. Mansonia

✓ **Ans:** B. Aedes

Q69. Measles elimination target year in India is:

◦ A. 2022
◦ B. 2023
◦ C. 2025
◦ D. 2030

✓ **Ans:** C. 2025

Q70. Skewed data has:
◦ A. Equal mean and median
◦ B. No mode
◦ C. Mean pulled in tail direction
◦ D. Median equals mode
✅ **Ans:** C. Mean pulled in tail direction

Q71. Which test has the **lowest false negatives**?
◦ A. Low sensitivity
◦ B. High specificity
◦ C. High sensitivity
◦ D. Low specificity
✅ **Ans:** C. High sensitivity

Q72. Which of the following shows a **bell-shaped curve**?
◦ A. Skewed data
◦ B. Bimodal distribution
◦ C. Normal distribution
◦ D. Logarithmic curve
✅ **Ans:** C. Normal distribution

Q73. BCG scar is formed due to:
◦ A. Killed mycobacteria
◦ B. Pyogenic reaction
◦ C. Delayed hypersensitivity
◦ D. Live attenuated toxin
✅ **Ans:** C. Delayed hypersensitivity

Q74. Time between infection and **becoming infectious** is called:
◦ A. Incubation period
◦ B. Latent period
◦ C. Serial interval
◦ D. Lead time
✅ **Ans:** B. Latent period

Q75. Correlation coefficient (r) ranges from:
◦ A. −2 to +2
◦ B. −1 to +1
◦ C. 0 to 100
◦ D. 0 to 1
✅ **Ans:** B. −1 to +1

Q76. Health education belongs to which prevention level?
◦ A. Primordial
◦ B. Primary
◦ C. Secondary
◦ D. Tertiary
✅ **Ans:** B. Primary

Q77.
Disposal method for **expired cytotoxic drugs**:
◦ A. Incineration
◦ B. Autoclave
◦ C. Deep burial
◦ D. Shredding
✅ **Ans:** A. Incineration

Q78. Standard deviation measures:
◦ A. Central tendency
◦ B. Error margin
◦ C. Spread of data
◦ D. Association
✅ **Ans:** C. Spread of data

Q79. A nurse gives polio drops at home during pulse polio. This is:
◦ A. Passive surveillance
◦ B. Active surveillance
◦ C. Sentinel surveillance
◦ D. Universal surveillance
✅ **Ans:** B. Active surveillance

Q80. Case detection by **mass survey** is an example of:
◦ A. Passive surveillance

◦ B. Active surveillance
◦ C. Sentinel reporting
◦ D. Secondary prevention
✅ **Ans:** B. Active surveillance

Q81.
Which disease has the **shortest incubation period**?
◦ A. Cholera
◦ B. Hepatitis A
◦ C. Measles
◦ D. Tetanus
✅ **Ans:** A. Cholera
Few hours to 5 days — often foodborne outbreak clue

Q82. Which test detects **TB antigen and Rif resistance**?
◦ A. Mantoux
◦ B. BACTEC
◦ C. CBNAAT (GeneXpert)
◦ D. Chest X-ray
✅ **Ans:** C. CBNAAT

Q83. ASHA is appointed at the ratio of:
◦ A. 1 per 500
◦ B. 1 per 1000
◦ C. 1 per 5000
◦ D. 1 per 10,000
✅ **Ans:** B. 1 per 1000 rural population

Q84. Yellow bag BMW is treated by:
◦ A. Incineration
◦ B. Shredding
◦ C. Chemical treatment
◦ D. Deep burial
✅ **Ans:** A. Incineration

Q85. Effectiveness of a vaccine is measured in:
◦ A. Trial
◦ B. Laboratory
◦ C. Community
◦ D. Animal model
✅ **Ans:** C. Community

Q86. Which of the following is **not a live vaccine**?
◦ A. Rotavirus
◦ B. MMR
◦ C. Hepatitis B
◦ D. BCG
✅ **Ans:** C. Hepatitis B

Q87. A disease is **eliminated** when:
◦ A. No new cases globally
◦ B. No new cases locally
◦ C. Reduced to sporadic cases
◦ D. No mortality
✅ **Ans:** B. No new cases locally
Eradication = global; elimination = geographic area

Q88.
All are waterborne except:
◦ A. Typhoid
◦ B. Hepatitis E
◦ C. Polio
◦ D. TB
✅ **Ans:** D. TB

Q89. RBSK includes screening for how many conditions?
◦ A. 2
◦ B. 4
◦ C. 6
◦ D. 10
✅ **Ans:** B. 4Ds (Defects, Diseases, Deficiencies, Developmental delays)

Q90. Hepatitis B vaccine is given via:
◦ A. IM, anterolateral thigh

◦ B. IM, deltoid
◦ C. Subcut, gluteal
◦ D. Oral

✅ **Ans:** A. IM, anterolateral thigh (in infants)

Q91. Most appropriate study design for **vaccine efficacy** in real-world settings?
◦ A. Case-control
◦ B. Cohort
◦ C. RCT
◦ D. Community trial

✅ **Ans:** B. Cohort

Q92. Which of the following is used to **compare two proportions**?
◦ A. Chi-square
◦ B. t-test
◦ C. ANOVA
◦ D. Z-test

✅ **Ans:** A. Chi-square

Q93.
Mode of transmission of **Kyasanur Forest Disease (KFD)**:
◦ A. Tick bite
◦ B. Mosquito bite
◦ C. Aerosol
◦ D. Rat urine

✅ **Ans:** A. Tick bite

Q94. Which test is used for **interobserver agreement**?
◦ A. Kappa statistic
◦ B. Chi-square
◦ C. t-test
◦ D. ANOVA

✅ **Ans:** A. Kappa statistic

Q95.
Which of the following is used for **assessing vaccine potency**?
◦ A. VVM
◦ B. Vial label
◦ C. Freeze tag
◦ D. Ice pack

✅ **Ans:** A. Vaccine Vial Monitor (VVM)

Q96.
NRHM was launched in:
◦ A. 2000
◦ B. 2003
◦ C. 2005
◦ D. 2008

✅ **Ans:** C. 2005

Q97.
Tertiary prevention aims to:
◦ A. Treat symptoms
◦ B. Restore function
◦ C. Prevent exposure
◦ D. Promote screening

✅ **Ans:** B. Restore function

Q98.
Which vaccine is given as a **birth dose** under UIP?
◦ A. Measles
◦ B. DPT
◦ C. Hepatitis B
◦ D. Rotavirus

✅ **Ans:** C. Hepatitis B

Q99.
Under JSY, who gets the **cash benefit**?
◦ A. ASHA
◦ B. Pregnant woman
◦ C. Doctor

◦ D. Nurse

✅ **Ans:** B. Pregnant woman

ASHA gets an incentive under separate provision

Q100.

Which mosquito breeds in **artificial containers**?

◦ A. Culex

◦ B. Aedes

◦ C. Mansonia

◦ D. Anopheles

✅ **Ans:** B. Aedes

Rapidfire One-Liners & Fact Sheets – PSM

Health Indicators

- • Best overall indicator of health: Infant Mortality Rate (IMR)
- • Most sensitive index of community health: Under-5 Mortality Rate
- • Maternal Mortality Ratio (MMR) – number of maternal deaths per 100,000 live births
- • Neonatal mortality: death within 28 days of birth
- • Perinatal mortality includes late fetal + early neonatal deaths
- • Dependency ratio = Population aged <15 + >65 / Population 15–64

Types of Studies in Epidemiology

Type	Description	Example
Cross-sectional	Snapshot at one point in time	KAP study, Prevalence survey
Case-control	Retrospective, compares cases vs controls	Smoking and lung cancer
Cohort	Prospective, compares exposed vs non-exposed	Smoking and future outcomes
RCT	Random allocation of intervention	Drug trials

Incubation Periods – Rapid Recall

- • Measles: 10 days to fever, 14 days to rash
- • Hepatitis A: 15–50 days (avg 28)
- • Rabies: 1–3 months (range: 9 days to >1 year)
- • Tetanus: 3–21 days
- • Chickenpox: 10–21 days

Vaccines – Key Classifications

Vaccine Type	Examples
Live Attenuated	BCG, OPV, Measles, Yellow Fever
Killed/Inactivated	IPV, Hepatitis A, Rabies
Toxoid	DPT (Tetanus, Diphtheria)
Subunit/Conjugate	Hib, Pneumococcal, HPV

Screening Tests – Key Facts

- • Sensitivity: Ability to detect true positives
- • Specificity: Ability to detect true negatives
- • PPV (Positive Predictive Value): Probability that a positive result is truly positive

- • NPV (Negative Predictive Value): Probability that a negative result is truly negative
- • Gold standard for screening evaluation: ROC curve
- • Best test for ruling out disease: High Sensitivity (SnNOut)
- • Best test for ruling in disease: High Specificity (SpPIn)

Levels of Prevention – Summary Table

Level	Definition	Example
Primordial	Prevention of risk factor emergence	Discouraging junk food in children
Primary	Prevent onset of disease	Immunization, Health education
Secondary	Early diagnosis & treatment	Screening for hypertension, Pap smear
Tertiary	Reduce complications & disability	Rehabilitation for stroke
Quaternary	Avoid over-medicalization	Avoiding unnecessary investigations

National Health Programs – Key Highlights

- • RCH Program covers RMNCH+A (Reproductive, Maternal, Newborn, Child and Adolescent Health)
- • Mission Indradhanush: Aims to increase full immunization coverage
- • Janani Suraksha Yojana (JSY): Conditional cash transfer for institutional delivery
- • RNTCP (now NTEP): DOTS strategy for TB control
- • NPCDCS: Targets diabetes, hypertension, cancer
- • IDSP: Integrated Disease Surveillance Programme for early detection of outbreaks

Epidemiological Definitions – Must Know

- • Endemic: Constant presence of a disease in a population
- • Epidemic: Sudden increase in disease cases above normal
- • Pandemic: Epidemic spread across countries/continents
- • Sporadic: Occasional, irregular disease occurrence
- • Incidence: New cases in a population over a time period
- • Prevalence: All existing cases at a point in time
- • Attack rate: Proportion of exposed who develop disease
- • Case fatality rate: Deaths among diagnosed cases

Modes of Disease Transmission

Mode of Transmission	Examples
Direct contact	STDs, Leprosy

Droplet	Influenza, Diphtheria, COVID-19
Vector-borne	Malaria, Dengue, Filariasis
Vehicle-borne	Hepatitis A (water), Food poisoning
Airborne	TB, Measles, Varicella
Fomite	MRSA, Conjunctivitis
Transplacental	HIV, Rubella, Syphilis

Nutrition Programs – Essentials

- • Mid-Day Meal Scheme: Hot cooked meals in schools to improve nutrition and attendance
- • ICDS: Integrated Child Development Services – Anganwadi based, covers children <6 yrs and mothers
- • NNAPP: National Nutrition Anaemia Prophylaxis Program – Iron-folic acid for children and women
- • Vitamin A Prophylaxis: 9 doses from 9 months to 5 years
- • POSHAN Abhiyaan: India's flagship nutrition mission focusing on children, pregnant women and lactating mothers

International Health Agencies – Snapshot

Agency	Headquarters	Function / Role
WHO	Geneva, Switzerland	Global health leadership and technical support
UNICEF	New York, USA	Child health and welfare
UNFPA	New York, USA	Population and reproductive health
World Bank	Washington D.C., USA	Funding development and health programs
FAO	Rome, Italy	Food security and agriculture

Health Planning in India – Timeline Highlights

- • First Five-Year Plan (1951–56): Focused on agriculture and community development
- • Second Plan: Emphasized industrial development and health infrastructure
- • Bhore Committee recommendations formed the basis of early plans
- • 12th Five-Year Plan (2012–17): Last official plan before NITI Aayog model
- • NITI Aayog (2015): Replaced Planning Commission, promotes cooperative federalism
- • National Health Policy 2017: Aims at universal health coverage

Miscellaneous Must-Know Facts

- • DALY = YLL (Years of Life Lost) + YLD (Years Lived with Disability)
- • Health education: Most effective method for behavioral change – Personal communication

- • Safe delivery kit under: Janani Suraksha Yojana
- • ASHA workers: One per 1000 population in rural areas
- • Triage color coding: Red – Immediate, Yellow – Delayed, Green – Minor, Black – Dead
- • Herd immunity threshold varies per disease (e.g. Measles > 95%)

Pathology PYQs for NEET PG

Q1. A 40-year-old man has generalized lymphadenopathy. LN biopsy shows Reed–Sternberg cells that are CD15+ and CD30+. Diagnosis?
A. Non-Hodgkin lymphoma
B. Classical Hodgkin lymphoma
C. Anaplastic large cell lymphoma
D. T-cell lymphoma
✅ **Ans:** B. Classical Hodgkin lymphoma
Tip: *"15 × 2 = 30" = Classic HL markers*

Q2. A 7-year-old child has abdominal mass. Biopsy: starry-sky appearance. t(8;14) seen. Most likely diagnosis?
A. Follicular lymphoma
B. Burkitt lymphoma
C. DLBCL
D. LCH
✅ **Ans:** B. Burkitt lymphoma
Key Concept: c-MYC translocation → rapid turnover → apoptotic debris → starry sky

---

Q3. A patient with anemia shows ringed sideroblasts in bone marrow. Likely diagnosis?
A. Megaloblastic anemia
B. Iron deficiency anemia
C. Sideroblastic anemia
D. Hemolytic anemia
✅ **Ans:** C. Sideroblastic anemia
Clue: Prussian blue stain detects iron-laden mitochondria

Q4. Which of the following is seen in Hairy Cell Leukemia?
A. Smudge cells
B. Reed–Sternberg cells
C. TRAP positivity
D. Dutcher bodies
✅ **Ans:** C. TRAP positivity
☐ Also CD11c+, CD25+

Q5. t(15;17) is associated with?
A. CML
B. AML-M3
C. ALL
D. CLL
✅ **Ans:** B. AML-M3 (APML)
Life-threatening DIC risk → treat with ATRA

Q6. Which of the following stains amyloid?
A. Masson trichrome
B. Congo red
C. PAS
D. Giemsa
✅ **Ans:** B. Congo red
Shows **apple-green birefringence** under polarized light

Q7. Target cells are seen in all except:
A. Thalassemia
B. Liver disease
C. HbC disease
D. Iron deficiency anemia
✅ **Ans:** D. Iron deficiency anemia
Mnemonic: **"THaL** has target cells" – **T**halassemia, **H**bC, **L**iver disease

Q8. CD markers for Classical Hodgkin Lymphoma?
A. CD3 and CD20
B. CD15 and CD30
C. CD10 and CD19
D. CD5 and CD23
✅ **Ans:** B. CD15 and CD30

Q9. Starry-sky appearance seen in which lymphoma?
✅ **Ans:** Burkitt lymphoma

Q10. A patient is on methotrexate. His blood smear shows macrocytic anemia with hypersegmented neutrophils. Most likely deficiency?
✅ **Ans:** Folic acid

Q11. A 65-year-old man presents with fatigue and lymphadenopathy. Smear shows small mature lymphocytes with smudge cells. CD5+, CD23+. Likely diagnosis?
A. AML
B. CML
C. CLL
D. Hairy cell leukemia
✅ **Ans:** C. Chronic Lymphocytic Leukemia
Mnemonic: *"Old man + Smudge cells = CLL"*
Markers: **CD5+, CD23+** (B-cell malignancy)

Q12. Philadelphia chromosome t(9;22) is diagnostic of:
A. CML
B. ALL
C. AML
D. CLL
✅ **Ans:** A. CML
Explanation: BCR-ABL fusion gene → ↑ tyrosine kinase activity → treat with **Imatinib**

Q13. A patient with fatigue and bone pain has lytic bone lesions. Serum protein electrophoresis shows M spike. Likely diagnosis?
A. AML
B. Hodgkin lymphoma
C. Multiple myeloma
D. CLL
✅ **Ans:** C. Multiple Myeloma
Features: CRAB (Calcium↑, Renal failure, Anemia, Bone lesions)

Q14. Apple-green birefringence on Congo red stain is diagnostic of:
A. Lipofuscin
B. Amyloid
C. Iron
D. Hemosiderin
✅ **Ans:** B. Amyloid

Q15. Bone marrow shows dry tap in a patient with pancytopenia. Most likely diagnosis:
A. CML
B. AML
C. Hairy Cell Leukemia
D. Multiple Myeloma
✅ **Ans:** C. Hairy Cell Leukemia
Explanation: Cells get trapped in reticulin mesh → **dry tap** on aspiration
Markers: CD11c+, CD25+, TRAP+

Q16. A young adult has enlarged lymph nodes. LN biopsy shows large cells with "owl eye" nucleoli, CD15+, CD30+. Most likely diagnosis?

✅ **Ans:** Classical Hodgkin Lymphoma
Reed–Sternberg cells = diagnostic

Q17. Which of the following is a tumor suppressor gene?
A. RAS
B. p53
C. MYC
D. BCL2

✅ **Ans:** B. p53
"Guardian of the genome" – regulates apoptosis; mutated in many cancers

Q18. Micronodular cirrhosis is characteristic of:
A. Alcoholic liver disease
B. Hemochromatosis
C. Wilson's disease
D. HBV infection

✅ **Ans:** A. Alcoholic liver disease
Repeated injury → regenerative small nodules

Q19. Pautrier microabscesses in skin biopsy indicate:
A. Psoriasis
B. Pemphigus
C. Mycosis fungoides
D. Dermatitis herpetiformis

✅ **Ans:** C. Mycosis fungoides
T-cell cutaneous lymphoma; Pautrier = intraepidermal clusters of lymphocytes

Q20. A 28-year-old female presents with pancytopenia. Bone marrow is hypocellular with fatty replacement. Diagnosis?

✅ **Ans:** Aplastic Anemia
Often idiopathic, drug-induced, or post-viral
Monitor for infections, bleeding

Format: Clinical recall + explanation + memory pearls

Q21. A patient presents with progressive fatigue. Bone marrow shows >20% blasts positive for MPO. Diagnosis?
A. ALL
B. AML
C. CML
D. CLL

✅ **Ans:** B. Acute Myeloid Leukemia
>20% blasts + **MPO positivity** = AML
Auer rods may be seen

Q22. Which stain is used to detect iron in bone marrow?
A. PAS
B. Sudan black
C. Giemsa
D. Prussian blue

✅ **Ans:** D. Prussian Blue
Detects ferric iron – **used in sideroblastic anemia**

Q23. Which one of the following is not an oncogene?
A. RAS
B. p53
C. MYC
D. ABL

✅ **Ans:** B. p53
p53 = tumor suppressor, others are oncogenes

Q24. Dutcher bodies are seen in:
A. AML

B. Multiple myeloma
C. Waldenström macroglobulinemia
D. Hairy cell leukemia

✅ **Ans:** C. Waldenström macroglobulinemia

Explanation: Dutcher bodies = intranuclear inclusions of IgM

Q25. Reed–Sternberg cells are seen in:
A. Burkitt lymphoma
B. Follicular lymphoma
C. Hodgkin lymphoma
D. Multiple myeloma

✅ **Ans:** C. Hodgkin lymphoma

CD15+, CD30+, Owl-eye nucleus

Q26. A patient presents with sudden onset hematuria. Urine shows RBC casts. Renal biopsy shows subepithelial humps. Most likely diagnosis?
A. RPGN
B. Minimal change disease
C. Post-streptococcal GN
D. Membranous GN

✅ **Ans:** C. Post-streptococcal GN

Key word: *"humps" = immune complex deposits under epithelium*

Q27. Heinz bodies are best seen with:
A. PAS
B. Giemsa
C. Supravital stain
D. Reticulin stain

✅ **Ans:** C. Supravital stain

Used for G6PD deficiency screening

Q28. Target cells are NOT seen in:
A. Thalassemia
B. Liver disease
C. Iron deficiency anemia
D. HbC disease

✅ **Ans:** C. Iron deficiency anemia

Seen in Thalassemia, HbC, Liver (THaL)

Q29. Which is a pre-malignant lesion?
A. Hyperplasia
B. Metaplasia
C. Dysplasia
D. Anaplasia

✅ **Ans:** C. Dysplasia

Can progress to carcinoma in situ

Q30. G6PD deficiency leads to:
A. Extravascular hemolysis
B. Intravascular hemolysis
C. Megaloblastic anemia
D. Hypoplastic anemia

✅ **Ans:** B. Intravascular hemolysis

Triggered by sulfa drugs, fava beans → Heinz bodies

Q31. Which of the following is a feature of apoptosis?
A. Inflammation
B. Cell lysis
C. DNA fragmentation
D. Cell swelling

✅ **Ans:** C. DNA fragmentation

Apoptosis: cell shrinkage, **membrane blebbing**, and DNA laddering

No inflammation → unlike necrosis

Q32. A patient presents with hepatosplenomegaly and anemia. Bone marrow shows Gaucher cells. Diagnosis?
A. Niemann–Pick disease
B. Gaucher disease
C. Tay–Sachs disease
D. Fabry disease

✅ **Ans:** B. Gaucher disease

Gaucher cells = **"wrinkled tissue paper" cytoplasm**
Deficiency: β-glucocerebrosidase

Q33. Which enzyme is deficient in Pompe's disease?
A. Glucose-6-phosphatase
B. α-1,4-glucosidase
C. Galactose-1-P uridyltransferase
D. Hexosaminidase A

✅ **Ans:** B. α-1,4-glucosidase
Leads to glycogen accumulation in **heart and liver**
Pompe = *"Pump problem"* (heart)

Q34. Which of the following cells shows Auer rods?
A. Myeloblast
B. Lymphoblast
C. Plasma cell
D. Reticulocyte

✅ **Ans:** A. Myeloblast
☐ Found in AML, especially **M3 (APML)** subtype

Q35. "Owl eye" nucleus is seen in:
A. CMV
B. Hodgkin lymphoma
C. Herpes
D. Both A and B

✅ **Ans:** D. Both CMV and Hodgkin lymphoma
Reed–Sternberg cells (CD15+, CD30+)
CMV → inclusions resemble owl-eye

Q36. What is the histologic feature of papillary carcinoma thyroid?
A. Psammoma bodies
B. Spindle cells
C. Clear cells
D. Reed–Sternberg cells

✅ **Ans:** A. Psammoma bodies
Also: **Orphan Annie nuclei**, nuclear grooves
Papillary = Psammoma

Q37. Bence-Jones proteins are detected in:
A. ALL
B. CLL
C. Multiple myeloma
D. Hodgkin lymphoma

✅ **Ans:** C. Multiple Myeloma
Light chains (kappa or lambda) → **excreted in urine**

Q38. Flame cells are seen in:
A. Plasma cell myeloma
B. Hodgkin lymphoma
C. Burkitt lymphoma
D. Megaloblastic anemia

✅ **Ans:** A. Plasma cell myeloma
Plasma cells with red-staining cytoplasm due to immunoglobulins

---

Q39. Which of the following is a feature of CML?
A. Smudge cells
B. Basophilia
C. Rouleaux formation
D. Auer rods

✅ **Ans:** B. Basophilia
CML hallmark: ↑ **basophils + neutrophilic left shift + low LAP**

Q40. Marker for endothelial origin of tumor:
A. Cytokeratin
B. CD45
C. CD34
D. CD31

✅ **Ans:** D. CD31
CD31 = **PECAM-1**, specific for endothelial tumors (e.g., angiosarcoma)

Q41. Which protein is deposited in primary amyloidosis?
A. β2-microglobulin
B. Serum amyloid A
C. AL (light chains)
D. Transthyretin
✅ **Ans:** C. AL (light chains)
From plasma cell dyscrasias like **multiple myeloma**

Q42. Which is true about necrosis?
A. Requires ATP
B. Involves DNA laddering
C. Causes inflammation
D. Cell shrinks
✅ **Ans:** C. Causes inflammation
Unlike apoptosis, necrosis leads to membrane rupture → inflammatory response

---

Q43. Auer rods are composed of:
A. DNA
B. RNA
C. Azurophilic granules
D. Myelin
✅ **Ans:** C. Azurophilic granules
Found in **AML**, especially M3 subtype

Q44. In iron deficiency anemia, the reticulocyte count is:
A. Increased
B. Decreased
C. Normal
D. Variable
✅ **Ans:** B. Decreased
Reticulocyte response is blunted due to lack of iron for erythropoiesis

---

Q45. Which enzyme is deficient in Niemann–Pick disease?
A. Glucocerebrosidase
B. Sphingomyelinase
C. Hexosaminidase A
D. G6PD
✅ **Ans:** B. Sphingomyelinase
Leads to accumulation of sphingomyelin in **liver, spleen, CNS**
"No man picks his nose with his sphinger" = Niemann–Pick → Sphingomyelin

---

Q46. Which of the following shows hypersegmented neutrophils?
A. Aplastic anemia
B. Megaloblastic anemia
C. Iron deficiency anemia
D. Thalassemia
✅ **Ans:** B. Megaloblastic anemia
Vit B12 or folate deficiency → defective DNA synthesis

Q47. Most specific marker for epithelial origin of tumors:
A. CD45
B. Vimentin
C. Desmin
D. Cytokeratin
✅ **Ans:** D. Cytokeratin
Cytokeratin = epithelial
Desmin = muscle, CD45 = leukocyte, Vimentin = mesenchyme

Q48. Which of the following is a feature of chronic inflammation?
A. Neutrophils

B. Fibrinoid necrosis
C. Macrophages and lymphocytes
D. Edema

✅ **Ans:** C. Macrophages and lymphocytes
Chronic inflammation = mononuclear cells + fibrosis

Q49. Which of the following leads to microcytic hypochromic anemia?
A. Vitamin B12 deficiency
B. Folate deficiency
C. Iron deficiency
D. Aplastic anemia

✅ **Ans:** C. Iron deficiency
Iron ↓ → Hb ↓ → microcytic RBCs
Macrocytic = B12/folate

Q50. Which cell is the precursor of a macrophage?
A. Monocyte
B. Neutrophil
C. Basophil
D. Eosinophil

✅ **Ans:** A. Monocyte
Monocytes circulate in blood → enter tissue → become macrophages

---

Focus: Classic repeats, old-but-gold concepts, clinical twist

---

Q51. A 2-year-old child presents with hepatosplenomegaly and cherry-red spot in the macula. Diagnosis?
A. Gaucher disease
B. Tay–Sachs disease
C. Niemann–Pick disease
D. Fabry disease

✅ **Ans:** C. Niemann–Pick disease
Mnemonic: "No man picks with a cherry" → **Cherry red spot + sphingomyelinase deficiency**

Q52. A patient has ↑ serum ferritin, ↑ serum iron, ↓ TIBC. Most likely condition?
A. Iron deficiency anemia
B. Thalassemia
C. Hemochromatosis
D. Sideroblastic anemia

✅ **Ans:** C. Hemochromatosis
Iron overload pattern
"Bronze diabetes" – skin pigmentation + diabetes + cirrhosis

Q53. What stain is used for mucin in adenocarcinomas?
A. Congo red
B. Sudan black
C. PAS
D. Mucicarmine

✅ **Ans:** D. Mucicarmine
Highlights epithelial mucin – especially used in **adenocarcinomas**

Q54. Which is a feature of coagulative necrosis?
A. Seen in brain
B. Cellular architecture preserved initially
C. Liquefaction of tissues
D. Presence of granulomas

✅ **Ans:** B. Cellular architecture preserved
Seen in ischemic injury except **brain** (which shows liquefactive)

Q55. Which cell type is predominant in granulomas?
A. Neutrophils
B. Lymphocytes

C. Epithelioid macrophages
D. Plasma cells
✅ **Ans:** C. Epithelioid macrophages
Aggregates of activated macrophages + multinucleated giant cells

---

Q56. In multiple myeloma, cause of renal failure is:
A. Amyloid deposition
B. Hypercalcemia
C. Bence-Jones protein cast nephropathy
D. Obstructive uropathy
✅ **Ans:** C. Bence-Jones protein cast nephropathy
Light chains precipitate in tubules → cast nephropathy

Q57. Russell bodies are seen in:
A. Langerhans cell histiocytosis
B. Hairy cell leukemia
C. Plasma cells
D. Lymphoblasts
✅ **Ans:** C. Plasma cells
Eosinophilic immunoglobulin inclusions in plasma cell cytoplasm

---

Q58. Warthin–Finkeldey giant cells are found in:
A. Measles
B. Tuberculosis
C. Sarcoidosis
D. SLE
✅ **Ans:** A. Measles
Mnemonic: "Warthin is watching measles" – large multinucleated cells in lymphoid tissues

---

Q59. Which of the following tumors arises from blood vessels?
A. Schwannoma
B. Lipoma
C. Angiosarcoma
D. Leiomyoma
✅ **Ans:** C. Angiosarcoma
CD31+ → endothelial tumor; seen in **liver, post-radiation**

Q60. What is the earliest change seen in reversible cell injury?
A. Nuclear pyknosis
B. Cell membrane rupture
C. Mitochondrial swelling
D. Karyorrhexis
✅ **Ans:** C. Mitochondrial swelling
Due to **failure of Na^+/K^+ pump** → water influx

Focus: Immunohistochemistry, renal/liver/lung pathology, image-based recall

---

Q61. Which immunohistochemical marker is positive in mesenchymal tumors?
A. Cytokeratin
B. Vimentin
C. CD45
D. CD31
✅ **Ans:** B. Vimentin
Marker for **mesenchymal origin** – sarcomas
Cytokeratin = epithelial, CD45 = leukocytes, CD31 = endothelial

---

Q62. Which of the following is seen in minimal change disease?
A. Subepithelial deposits
B. Fusion of foot processes on EM
C. Granular deposits
D. Crescents
✅ **Ans:** B. Fusion of foot processes

Most common nephrotic syndrome in children
Light microscopy = normal
Electron microscopy = **effacement of podocytes**

Q63. Which renal condition shows "wire loop" lesions on LM?
A. Diabetic nephropathy
B. Post-strep GN
C. Lupus nephritis
D. IgA nephropathy
✅ **Ans:** C. Lupus nephritis
Due to **immune complex deposition** in subendothelial region

---

Q64. Which pattern of necrosis is classically seen in brain infarct?
A. Coagulative
B. Caseous
C. Liquefactive
D. Fat
✅ **Ans:** C. Liquefactive necrosis
Enzymatic digestion + loss of tissue architecture

Q65. Which lung disease shows ferruginous bodies?
A. Coal workers' pneumoconiosis
B. Asbestosis
C. Silicosis
D. Hypersensitivity pneumonitis
✅ **Ans:** B. Asbestosis
Iron-coated asbestos fibers = **ferruginous bodies**

Q66. Psammoma bodies are seen in all except:
A. Papillary carcinoma thyroid
B. Meningioma
C. Serous cystadenocarcinoma ovary
D. Medullary thyroid carcinoma
✅ **Ans:** D. Medullary thyroid carcinoma
Psammoma: Papillary thyroid, Meningioma, Serous ovary, Mesothelioma
Mnemonic: "PSaMMoma" – all have double M

Q67. CD10 positivity is seen in:
A. Burkitt lymphoma
B. Follicular lymphoma
C. Mantle cell lymphoma
D. Marginal zone lymphoma
✅ **Ans:** B. Follicular lymphoma
t(14;18), BCL2 overexpression
CD10 = germinal center marker

Q68. A breast biopsy shows ducts filled with atypical cells, no invasion. Diagnosis?
A. DCIS
B. LCIS
C. Invasive ductal carcinoma
D. Inflammatory carcinoma
✅ **Ans:** A. Ductal Carcinoma In Situ (DCIS)
BM intact = **in situ**
Image-based question with **microcalcifications**

Q69. CD117 (c-Kit) is a marker for:
A. Neuroblastoma
B. GIST
C. Melanoma
D. Ewing's sarcoma
✅ **Ans:** B. Gastrointestinal Stromal Tumor (GIST)
Treated with **Imatinib** (tyrosine kinase inhibitor)

Q70. Which type of cell is most commonly involved in sarcoidosis granulomas?
A. Neutrophils
B. Plasma cells
C. Epithelioid histiocytes
D. Langerhans cells
✅ **Ans:** C. Epithelioid histiocytes
Sarcoid = **non-caseating granulomas**
Also see **Schaumann and asteroid bodies**

Focus: Blood groups, anemia clues, coagulation disorders, marrow changes

---

Q71. Which of the following blood groups is universal donor?
A. AB+
B. AB−
C. O−
D. O+
✅ **Ans:** C. O−
No A/B antigens, and Rh− avoids sensitization
Universal recipient = AB+

Q72. Which anemia shows increased RDW and hypersegmented neutrophils?
A. Thalassemia
B. Megaloblastic anemia
C. Sideroblastic anemia
D. Anemia of chronic disease
✅ **Ans:** B. Megaloblastic anemia
Vit B12/Folate deficiency
High MCV + oval macrocytes + neutrophil hypersegmentation

Q73. A patient with chronic blood loss has microcytic hypochromic anemia. Likely lab findings?
A. ↓ Serum ferritin, ↑ TIBC
B. ↑ Ferritin, ↓ TIBC
C. ↑ Serum iron
D. ↑ MCV
✅ **Ans:** A. ↓ Serum ferritin, ↑ TIBC
Iron deficiency anemia labs
Ferritin ↓ = stores depleted
TIBC ↑ = liver trying to grab more iron

Q74. Which of the following is best indicator of recent RBC production?
A. Reticulocyte count
B. Hemoglobin
C. Hematocrit
D. MCV
✅ **Ans:** A. Reticulocyte count
Retics = young RBCs → ↑ in hemolysis or post-therapy recovery

---

Q75. Which of the following tests is used to monitor warfarin therapy?
A. aPTT
B. PT/INR
C. Bleeding time
D. Thrombin time
✅ **Ans:** B. PT/INR
Warfarin affects **extrinsic pathway** (factors II, VII, IX, X, protein C/S)

Q76. Which clotting factor is vitamin K dependent?
A. Factor VIII
B. Factor V
C. Factor II
D. Factor XII
✅ **Ans:** C. Factor II
Vit K dependent: **2, 7, 9, 10, C, S**
Blocked by warfarin

Q77. Which is the earliest hematologic abnormality in iron deficiency anemia?
A. Low MCH
B. Low MCV
C. Low serum ferritin
D. High RDW

✅ **Ans:** C. Low serum ferritin

Ferritin drops first before MCV/MCH fall

Q78. Howell–Jolly bodies are seen in:
A. Iron deficiency anemia
B. Sickle cell anemia
C. Aplastic anemia
D. Megaloblastic anemia

✅ **Ans:** B. Sickle cell anemia

Due to **autosplenectomy** → nuclear remnants not cleared

Q79. Which coagulation disorder shows prolonged aPTT but normal PT?
A. Hemophilia A
B. Vitamin K deficiency
C. Liver disease
D. DIC

✅ **Ans:** A. Hemophilia A

Factor VIII deficiency → **intrinsic pathway defect**

Q80. Which test is most sensitive for DIC?
A. PT
B. aPTT
C. D-dimer
D. Platelet count

✅ **Ans:** C. D-dimer

Fibrin degradation product – **best early marker**

Focus: TB, leprosy, cell injury, pigment disorders, viral inclusions

---

Q81. Caseating granulomas are most commonly associated with:
A. Sarcoidosis
B. Tuberculosis
C. Crohn's disease
D. Leprosy

✅ **Ans:** B. Tuberculosis

Granulomas with central necrosis
Ziehl–Neelsen stain for acid-fast bacilli

Q82. A patient with lepromatous leprosy shows which type of granuloma?
A. Caseating
B. Non-caseating
C. Poor granuloma formation
D. Giant cell granuloma

✅ **Ans:** C. Poor granuloma formation

Th2 response dominates → ineffective immunity
High bacillary load

Q83. Ghon complex refers to:
A. Reactivation TB lesion
B. Primary TB in upper lobe
C. Primary TB + lymph node involvement
D. TB cavity formation

✅ **Ans:** C. Primary TB + lymph node involvement

Ghon focus (subpleural) + LN = **Ghon complex**

Q84. Which pigment is derived from oxidation of tyrosine?
A. Lipofuscin
B. Hemosiderin
C. Melanin
D. Bilirubin

✅ **Ans:** C. Melanin

Tyrosinase → dopa → melanin
Produced by melanocytes

Q85. Which of the following is a hallmark of irreversible cell injury?
A. Cell swelling
B. Ribosomal detachment
C. Nuclear pyknosis
D. Decreased ATP
✅ **Ans:** C. Nuclear pyknosis
Followed by karyorrhexis → karyolysis
Also: **membrane damage** is irreversible

Q86. Which of the following is not seen in apoptosis?
A. Cell shrinkage
B. Inflammation
C. Caspase activation
D. Membrane blebbing
✅ **Ans:** B. Inflammation
Apoptosis = clean, programmed death
Necrosis = inflammation

Q87. A 60-year-old man with alcoholic cirrhosis has golden brown cytoplasmic pigment in liver. Likely pigment?
A. Bilirubin
B. Hemosiderin
C. Lipofuscin
D. Melanin
✅ **Ans:** B. Hemosiderin
Seen in **secondary hemosiderosis** due to chronic hemolysis or transfusion

---

Q88. Councilman bodies in liver biopsy indicate:
A. Apoptotic hepatocytes
B. Mallory bodies
C. Amyloid deposition
D. Fatty change
✅ **Ans:** A. Apoptotic hepatocytes
Seen in viral hepatitis
Round eosinophilic apoptotic cells

Q89. In fatty liver, which stain is most appropriate?
A. PAS
B. Sudan IV
C. Congo red
D. Giemsa
✅ **Ans:** B. Sudan IV
Stains **neutral lipids** – fat vacuoles in liver, atherosclerosis

---

Q90. In viral infections, which inclusion body is found in CMV?
A. Negri bodies
B. Owl eye inclusion
C. Henderson–Patterson bodies
D. Guarnieri bodies
✅ **Ans:** B. Owl eye inclusion
CMV = large nuclear and cytoplasmic inclusions
"CMV = Cytomegalo Virus = Big owl eyes"

Focus: Wrap-up recall, system path integration, final revision pearls

---

Q91. "Nutmeg liver" is seen in:
A. Cirrhosis
B. Chronic passive congestion of liver
C. Hemochromatosis
D. Fatty liver
✅ **Ans:** B. Chronic passive congestion
Due to right heart failure → congested central veins
Nutmeg appearance = mottled red & yellow

Q92. Which is the gold standard for iron stores in the body?
A. Serum iron
B. Serum ferritin
C. TIBC
D. Bone marrow iron stain
✅ **Ans:** D. Bone marrow iron stain
Prussian blue staining used

Q93. Libman–Sacks endocarditis is seen in:
A. Rheumatic fever
B. SLE
C. Infective endocarditis
D. Antiphospholipid syndrome
✅ **Ans:** B. SLE
Sterile vegetations on both sides of mitral/tricuspid valves

Q94. Which tumor is most radiosensitive?
A. Chondrosarcoma
B. Osteosarcoma
C. Ewing sarcoma
D. Giant cell tumor
✅ **Ans:** C. Ewing sarcoma
t(11;22), small round blue cells, onion-skinning on X-ray

Q95. What is the most common site of atherosclerotic plaque formation?
A. Coronary arteries
B. Carotid arteries
C. Abdominal aorta
D. Renal arteries
✅ **Ans:** C. Abdominal aorta
Most prone to plaque → aneurysm formation

Q96. A young female has mitral stenosis and Aschoff bodies on biopsy. Likely diagnosis?
A. Infective endocarditis
B. RHD
C. SLE
D. Pericarditis
✅ **Ans:** B. Rheumatic Heart Disease
Aschoff bodies = granulomatous lesions of myocardium

Q97. "Onion-skin" periosteal reaction is seen in:
A. Osteosarcoma
B. Chondrosarcoma
C. Ewing sarcoma
D. Fibrous dysplasia
✅ **Ans:** C. Ewing sarcoma

Q98. A patient has hematuria 5 days after URI. Likely diagnosis?
A. PSGN
B. IgA nephropathy
C. Minimal change disease
D. Lupus nephritis
✅ **Ans:** B. IgA nephropathy
Berger's disease – most common glomerulonephritis worldwide
Key clue: **within 1 week** of URI

Q99. Which of the following is a type of metaplasia?
A. Columnar to squamous in bronchi
B. Squamous to columnar in esophagus
C. Dysplasia of epithelium
D. Atrophy of muscle
✅ **Ans:** A. Columnar to squamous

Seen in chronic smoking – reversible adaptation

Q100. Which cell adaptation is seen in uterine enlargement during pregnancy?
A. Hyperplasia
B. Atrophy
C. Metaplasia
D. Hypertrophy

✅ **Ans:** D. Hypertrophy
Increase in **cell size**, not number
Occurs in **smooth muscle of uterus**

Revision Boost: 50 Bonus Pathology PYQs

Q1. Which interleukin is secreted by macrophages and causes fever?

◦ A. IL-2
◦ B. IL-1
◦ C. IL-10
◦ D. IL-12

✓ Ans: B. IL-1

Explanation: IL-1 = endogenous pyrogen; also activates T cells.

◦ A. IL-2
◦ B. IL-1
◦ C. IL-10
◦ D. IL-12

✓ Ans: B. IL-1

Explanation: IL-1 = endogenous pyrogen; also activates T cells.

Q2. CD34 is a marker for:

◦ A. Endothelial cells
◦ B. Plasma cells
◦ C. T cells
◦ D. Macrophages

✓ Ans: A. Endothelial cells

Explanation: Also a stem cell marker.

Q3. Pseudopalisading necrosis is seen in:

◦ A. Glioblastoma
◦ B. Medulloblastoma
◦ C. Oligodendroglioma
◦ D. Ependymoma

✓ Ans: A. Glioblastoma

Explanation: Central necrosis surrounded by tumor cells.

Q4. Russell bodies are:

◦ A. Nuclear remnants
◦ B. Mitochondrial inclusions
◦ C. Immunoglobulin accumulations
◦ D. Autophagic vacuoles

✓ Ans: C. Immunoglobulin accumulations

Explanation: Seen in plasma cells.

Q5. Which phase of wound healing involves macrophages?

◦ A. Hemostasis
◦ B. Inflammation
◦ C. Proliferation
◦ D. Maturation

✓ Ans: B. Inflammation

Explanation: Macrophages dominate after neutrophils (48–72 hrs).

Q6. Which of the following is not a feature of malignancy?

◦ A. Pleomorphism
◦ B. Hyperchromatism
◦ C. Loss of polarity
◦ D. Uniform nuclei

✓ Ans: D. Uniform nuclei

Explanation: Malignancy shows nuclear variability.

Q7. What type of necrosis is seen in pancreatitis?

◦ A. Coagulative
◦ B. Liquefactive
◦ C. Fat
◦ D. Caseous

✅ Ans: C. Fat
Explanation: Lipase-mediated fat saponification.

Q8. Amyloid in Alzheimer's disease is derived from:
◦ A. β2-microglobulin
◦ B. Aβ protein
◦ C. Transthyretin
◦ D. Immunoglobulin light chain
✅ Ans: B. Aβ protein
Explanation: Derived from amyloid precursor protein (APP).

Q9. Heinz bodies seen in:
◦ A. Sickle cell anemia
◦ B. G6PD deficiency
◦ C. Thalassemia
◦ D. Iron deficiency anemia
✅ Ans: B. G6PD deficiency
Explanation: Oxidized denatured Hb precipitates in RBCs.

Q10. Best marker for cell proliferation:
◦ A. Ki-67
◦ B. p53
◦ C. Cyclin D1
◦ D. BCL2
✅ Ans: A. Ki-67
Explanation: Present during all active phases of cell cycle.

✅ That's Q1–Q10 of your Revision Add-On (50 total).
Next up: Q11–Q20 includes more hematology, infections, and image recalls.
Shall I continue?

Awesome! Here's the next batch of your NEET PG Pathology Revision Add-On: Q11–Q20
🎁 Focus: Hematology, image-based clues, stains, marrow logic

Q11. Auer rods are composed of:
◦ A. Immunoglobulin
◦ B. RNA
◦ C. Azurophilic granules
◦ D. Lipid droplets
✅ Ans: C. Azurophilic granules
Explanation: Diagnostic of AML, especially M3 (APML).

Q12. Hypersegmented neutrophils suggest deficiency of:
◦ A. Iron
◦ B. Vitamin C
◦ C. Folate
◦ D. Zinc
✅ Ans: C. Folate
Explanation: Seen in megaloblastic anemia (folate > B12).

Q13. "Tennis racket" shaped cytoplasmic granules are:
◦ A. Birbeck granules
◦ B. Russell bodies
◦ C. Auer rods
◦ D. Howell-Jolly bodies
✅ Ans: A. Birbeck granules
Explanation: Seen in Langerhans Cell Histiocytosis (CD1a+, S100+).

Q14. TRAP positivity is diagnostic of:
◦ A. ALL
◦ B. CLL
◦ C. Hairy Cell Leukemia

◦ D. Hodgkin's

✅ Ans: C. Hairy Cell Leukemia

Explanation: Tartrate-resistant acid phosphatase. Also CD11c+, CD25+.

Q15. Which stain highlights basement membranes?

◦ A. PAS

◦ B. Giemsa

◦ C. Masson trichrome

◦ D. Congo red

✅ Ans: A. PAS

Explanation: Highlights glycogen and basement membranes. Also useful in fungi.

Q16. Flame cells are characteristic of:

◦ A. Hodgkin lymphoma

◦ B. Plasma cell myeloma

◦ C. ALL

◦ D. MALToma

✅ Ans: B. Plasma cell myeloma

Explanation: Ig-filled plasma cells stain pink → "flame-like".

Q17. Howell–Jolly bodies indicate absence of:

◦ A. Liver

◦ B. Bone marrow

◦ C. Spleen

◦ D. Lymph nodes

✅ Ans: C. Spleen

Explanation: Nuclear remnants in RBCs not cleared due to asplenia or splenectomy.

Q18. Which of the following causes pancytopenia with hypocellular marrow?

◦ A. Megaloblastic anemia

◦ B. Myelofibrosis

◦ C. Aplastic anemia

◦ D. CML

✅ Ans: C. Aplastic anemia

Explanation: Bone marrow failure with fatty replacement.

Q19. Psammoma bodies are not seen in:

◦ A. Papillary thyroid carcinoma

◦ B. Meningioma

◦ C. Serous cystadenocarcinoma ovary

◦ D. Medullary thyroid carcinoma

✅ Ans: D. Medullary thyroid carcinoma

Explanation: "PSaMMoma" — Psammoma seen in Papillary, Serous, Meningioma, Mesothelioma.

Q20. Schiller-Duval bodies are seen in:

◦ A. Embryonal carcinoma

◦ B. Teratoma

◦ C. Yolk sac tumor

◦ D. Seminoma

✅ Ans: C. Yolk sac tumor

Explanation: Look like glomeruli; associated with high AFP.

Q21. Tumor suppressor gene mutated in retinoblastoma:

◦ A. p53

◦ B. Rb

◦ C. BRCA1

◦ D. NF1

✅ Ans: B. Rb

Explanation: 2-hit hypothesis; regulates G1 → S transition.

Q22. Oncogene implicated in Burkitt lymphoma:

◦ A. MYC

◦ B. RAS

◦ C. ABL

◦ D. RET

✅ Ans: A. MYC
Explanation: t(8;14) translocation → c-MYC overexpression.

Q23. DNA viruses causing cancer include all EXCEPT:
◦ A. HPV
◦ B. EBV
◦ C. Hepatitis B
◦ D. HCV
✅ Ans: D. HCV
Explanation: HCV is RNA virus; HBV (DNA) is oncogenic.

Q24. Which viral inclusion is found in CMV infection?
◦ A. Negri bodies
◦ B. Owl-eye inclusions
◦ C. Henderson–Patterson bodies
◦ D. Guarnieri bodies
✅ Ans: B. Owl-eye inclusions
Explanation: Large eosinophilic intranuclear inclusion in cytomegalovirus.

Q25. p53 gene is located on which chromosome?
◦ A. 5
◦ B. 7
◦ C. 17
◦ D. 13
✅ Ans: C. Chromosome 17
Explanation: Mutated in Li-Fraumeni syndrome.

Q26. PAS-positive macrophages in lamina propria suggest:
◦ A. Crohn's disease
◦ B. Celiac disease
◦ C. Whipple disease
◦ D. TB
✅ Ans: C. Whipple disease
Explanation: Tropheryma whipplei — foamy macrophages with PAS-positive granules.

Q27. Hyaline membrane disease in neonates shows:
◦ A. Surfactant excess
◦ B. Alveolar hemorrhage
◦ C. Protein-rich membranes lining alveoli
◦ D. Atelectasis
✅ Ans: C. Protein-rich membranes lining alveoli
Explanation: Due to surfactant deficiency in preterm lungs.

Q28. "String sign" on barium study is classically seen in:
◦ A. Ulcerative colitis
◦ B. Crohn's disease
◦ C. Carcinoid
◦ D. Gastric ulcer
✅ Ans: B. Crohn's disease
Explanation: Severe narrowing of terminal ileum due to transmural inflammation.

Q29. Which of the following is an anti-apoptotic gene?
◦ A. p53
◦ B. Bax
◦ C. BCL-2
◦ D. Caspase
✅ Ans: C. BCL-2
Explanation: Overexpressed in follicular lymphoma (t14;18).

Q30. Nutmeg liver is a feature of:
◦ A. Hemochromatosis
◦ B. Chronic passive congestion
◦ C. Wilson disease
◦ D. Reye's syndrome

✅ Ans: B. Chronic passive congestion
Explanation: Seen in right heart failure → mottled liver with central congestion.

Q31. Non-caseating granulomas are seen in all EXCEPT:
◦ A. Sarcoidosis
◦ B. Crohn's disease
◦ C. Leprosy
◦ D. Berylliosis

✅ Ans: C. Leprosy
Explanation: Leprosy usually shows caseating granulomas (esp. in tuberculoid type).

Q32. "Target cells" are seen in:
◦ A. Thalassemia
◦ B. HbC disease
◦ C. Liver disease
◦ D. All of the above

✅ Ans: D. All of the above
Explanation: Target cells = "THaL" = Thalassemia, HbC, Liver.

Q33. Sideroblastic anemia is associated with:
◦ A. Ringed sideroblasts
◦ B. Low ferritin
◦ C. Decreased serum iron
◦ D. Normal TIBC

✅ Ans: A. Ringed sideroblasts
Explanation: Seen with iron-loaded mitochondria around nuclei. Prussian blue stain.

Q34. Heinz bodies are best seen with:
◦ A. Giemsa stain
◦ B. Prussian blue
◦ C. Supravital stain
◦ D. PAS

✅ Ans: C. Supravital stain
Explanation: Identifies denatured Hb in G6PD deficiency.

Q35. Red blood cell with multiple fine basophilic dots:
◦ A. Reticulocyte
◦ B. Heinz body
◦ C. Basophilic stippling
◦ D. Howell–Jolly body

✅ Ans: C. Basophilic stippling
Explanation: Seen in lead poisoning, thalassemia, sideroblastic anemia.

Q36. Stain used for amyloid detection:
◦ A. PAS
◦ B. Giemsa
◦ C. Congo red
◦ D. Sudan IV

✅ Ans: C. Congo red
Explanation: Shows apple-green birefringence under polarized light.

Q37. Best site for bone marrow biopsy:
◦ A. Sternum
◦ B. Tibia
◦ C. Iliac crest
◦ D. Femur

✅ Ans: C. Iliac crest

Explanation: Posterior superior iliac spine is safest and most common.

Q38. Starry-sky appearance on histology is seen in:
◦ A. Follicular lymphoma
◦ B. Hodgkin lymphoma
◦ C. Burkitt lymphoma
◦ D. CLL

✅ Ans: C. Burkitt lymphoma
Explanation: Due to high mitotic rate and interspersed macrophages.

Q39. What is the major chemoattractant for neutrophils?
◦ A. IL-2
◦ B. IL-6
◦ C. IL-8
◦ D. IL-10

✅ Ans: C. IL-8
Explanation: Neutrophil migration during acute inflammation.

Q40. Dohle bodies are seen in:
◦ A. Megaloblastic anemia
◦ B. Leukemoid reaction
◦ C. Malaria
◦ D. Sickle cell anemia

✅ Ans: B. Leukemoid reaction
Explanation: Pale blue inclusions in neutrophils, seen with toxic granules.

Q41. Which of the following is the most potent antigen-presenting cell?
◦ A. Macrophage
◦ B. Dendritic cell
◦ C. B cell
◦ D. Langerhans cell

✅ Ans: B. Dendritic cell
Explanation: Best APC, activates naïve T cells efficiently.

Q42. Stain used to identify fungi:
◦ A. Giemsa
◦ B. Methenamine silver
◦ C. Prussian blue
◦ D. Sudan III

✅ Ans: B. Methenamine silver
Explanation: Highlights fungal walls in black.

Q43. Reticulocyte count is increased in all except:
◦ A. Hemolysis
◦ B. Blood loss
◦ C. Iron deficiency anemia
◦ D. After B12 therapy

✅ Ans: C. Iron deficiency anemia
Explanation: No iron → no RBC production → low retic.

Q44. The best test for hereditary spherocytosis:
◦ A. Osmotic fragility test
◦ B. Coombs test
◦ C. G6PD enzyme level
◦ D. Schilling test

✅ Ans: A. Osmotic fragility test
Explanation: Spherocytes burst easily in hypotonic solution.

Q45. CD10 is positive in:
◦ A. Mantle cell lymphoma
◦ B. Burkitt lymphoma
◦ C. Follicular lymphoma
◦ D. CLL

✅ Ans: C. Follicular lymphoma
Explanation: CD10 = Germinal center marker; seen in FL, some B-ALL.

Q46. Which immunoglobulin is first formed after antigen exposure?
◦ A. IgA
◦ B. IgE
◦ C. IgM
◦ D. IgG
✅ Ans: C. IgM
Explanation: Primary immune response = IgM. Secondary = IgG.

Q47. Lipofuscin pigment is derived from:
◦ A. Iron
◦ B. Oxidized lipids
◦ C. Calcium
◦ D. Cholesterol
✅ Ans: B. Oxidized lipids
Explanation: "Wear and tear" pigment. Accumulates in elderly or cachexia.

Q48. Lead poisoning causes anemia due to inhibition of:
◦ A. Ferrochelatase and ALA dehydratase
◦ B. G6PD
◦ C. Glutathione synthetase
◦ D. ATP synthase
✅ Ans: A. Ferrochelatase and ALA dehydratase
Explanation: Causes microcytic anemia + basophilic stippling.

Q49. Waterhouse–Friderichsen syndrome is due to:
◦ A. Meningococcemia
◦ B. DIC
◦ C. EBV
◦ D. CMV
✅ Ans: A. Meningococcemia
Explanation: Hemorrhagic adrenal infarction + septic shock.

Q50. A cell with large, bilobed nucleus and bright red cytoplasmic granules is:
◦ A. Basophil
◦ B. Neutrophil
◦ C. Eosinophil
◦ D. Monocyte
✅ Ans: C. Eosinophil
Explanation: Seen in parasitic infections, allergies, Hodgkin's.

Pathology Key One liners, Tables & Facts

Types of Necrosis – Comparative Table

Type	Example	Microscopy
Coagulative	Myocardial infarction	Preserved architecture, eosinophilic cytoplasm
Liquefactive	Brain infarct, abscess	Loss of architecture, neutrophilic debris
Caseous	Tuberculosis (lungs)	Granular, cheesy necrotic debris
Fat	Acute pancreatitis, fat trauma	Chalky white areas, saponification
Fibrinoid	Vasculitis	Bright pink fibrin-like material in vessel wall

Inflammation Cell Types – Quick Reference

- • Neutrophils – Multilobed nucleus, acute inflammation
- • Eosinophils – Bilobed nucleus, red granules, allergies/parasitic infections
- • Macrophages – Kidney-shaped nucleus, chronic inflammation
- • Lymphocytes – Round nucleus, scant cytoplasm, viral infections/autoimmune
- • Plasma cells – Clock-face nucleus, chronic inflammation, antibody production

Cell Injury Markers – Organ Specific

Organ	Marker
Myocardium	Troponin I, CK-MB
Liver	AST, ALT, ALP, GGT
Pancreas	Amylase, Lipase
Skeletal muscle	CPK (MM), Aldolase

Hemodynamic Disorders – Essentials

- ◆ **Thrombosis – Virchow's Triad**
- - Endothelial injury
- - Abnormal blood flow (turbulence/stasis)
- - Hypercoagulability
- ◆ **Types of Embolism**
- • Thromboembolism – most common
- • Fat embolism – long bone fractures
- • Air embolism – decompression sickness, IV lines
- • Amniotic fluid embolism – during labor
- • Paradoxical embolism – venous clot enters arterial system via septal defect

Anemia Classification – Based on MCV

Type	MCV Range	Examples
Microcytic	< 80 fL	Iron deficiency, Thalassemia, Sideroblastic
Normocytic	80–100 fL	Hemolysis, Aplastic anemia, Chronic disease
Macrocytic	> 100 fL	Vitamin B12 or Folate deficiency, Liver disease

Important Stains & Their Uses

- • PAS – Glycogen, fungi (e.g., Candida)
- • Ziehl-Neelsen (ZN) – Acid-fast bacilli (Mycobacterium)
- • Congo Red – Amyloid (apple green birefringence under polarized light)
- • Giemsa – Malaria, Leishmania, H. pylori
- • Masson's Trichrome – Collagen (fibrosis detection)
- • Reticulin stain – Bone marrow architecture

WBC Disorders – Quick Reference

- • Neutrophilia – Bacterial infections, stress, steroids
- • Eosinophilia – Parasitic infections, allergies, Hodgkin's lymphoma
- • Lymphocytosis – Viral infections (EBV, CMV), CLL
- • Monocytosis – TB, chronic infections, monocytic leukemia
- • Basophilia – CML (Chronic Myeloid Leukemia)

Tumor Markers – Must-Know Associations

Marker	Associated Cancer
AFP	Hepatocellular carcinoma, Yolk sac tumor
CEA	Colorectal, pancreatic, gastric cancers
CA-125	Ovarian cancer
CA 19-9	Pancreatic cancer
PSA	Prostate cancer
β-hCG	Choriocarcinoma, germ cell tumors
Calcitonin	Medullary thyroid carcinoma

Genetic Inheritance Patterns – Table

Pattern	Description	Examples
Autosomal Dominant	Vertical transmission, both sexes affected	Marfan, Huntington’s, Familial hypercholesterolemia
Autosomal Recessive	Often skips generations, consanguinity	CF, Sickle cell anemia, Thalassemia
X-linked Recessive	More in males, mothers are carriers	Hemophilia A/B, G6PD deficiency, Duchenne MD

Mitochondrial	Maternal inheritance only	Leber's optic neuropathy

Microbiology PYQs for NEET PG

Q1. NEET PG 2024
A patient presents with a painless genital ulcer. Dark-field microscopy shows motile corkscrew organisms. Likely organism?
◦ A. Treponema pallidum
◦ B. Haemophilus ducreyi
◦ C. Klebsiella granulomatis
◦ D. Chlamydia trachomatis (L1–L3)
✅ Ans: A. Treponema pallidum
Explanation: Classic primary syphilis; diagnosed by dark-field microscopy. Motile spirochete.

Q2. NEET PG 2024
Which bacterial structure is used for conjugation?
◦ A. Fimbriae
◦ B. Flagella
◦ C. Pili (sex pilus)
◦ D. Capsule
✅ Ans: C. Pili (sex pilus)
Explanation: F+ plasmid → sex pilus formation → horizontal gene transfer via conjugation.

Q3. NEET PG 2024
A neonate develops meningitis. Gram stain shows gram-negative rods. Most likely organism?
◦ A. Streptococcus agalactiae
◦ B. E. coli
◦ C. Listeria monocytogenes
◦ D. HSV-2
✅ Ans: B. E. coli
Explanation: In neonates, E. coli (K1 strain) is a common cause of meningitis along with GBS and Listeria.

Q4. NEET PG 2024
Which virus is associated with temporal lobe hemorrhagic encephalitis?
◦ A. CMV
◦ B. HSV-1
◦ C. Rabies
◦ D. VZV
✅ Ans: B. HSV-1
Explanation: HSV-1 → necrotizing encephalitis with hemorrhage, especially temporal lobes.

Q5.
A patient with prolonged hospitalization and broad-spectrum antibiotics develops diarrhea. Stool ELISA is positive for a bacterial toxin. Most likely organism?
◦ A. Salmonella
◦ B. Clostridium perfringens
◦ C. Clostridium difficile
◦ D. Vibrio cholerae
✅ Ans: C. Clostridium difficile
Explanation: Antibiotic-associated colitis → Toxin A/B detection confirms C. difficile.

Q6.
Ziehl–Neelsen stain is used to detect:
◦ A. Mycoplasma
◦ B. Nocardia
◦ C. Cryptococcus
◦ D. Mycobacterium tuberculosis
✅ Ans: D. Mycobacterium tuberculosis

Explanation: Acid-fast stain detects mycolic acid in cell wall.

Q7.
A 6-year-old presents with fever, sore throat, and a gray membrane in throat. The organism is found to be gram-positive bacilli with metachromatic granules. Likely cause?
◦ A. Streptococcus pyogenes
◦ B. Corynebacterium diphtheriae
◦ C. Staphylococcus aureus
◦ D. Haemophilus influenzae
✅ Ans: B. Corynebacterium diphtheriae
Explanation: Characteristic pseudomembrane + Albert stain positive granules.

Q8.
All of the following are live attenuated vaccines EXCEPT:
◦ A. MMR
◦ B. BCG
◦ C. Hepatitis B
◦ D. OPV
✅ Ans: C. Hepatitis B
Explanation: Hepatitis B = recombinant subunit vaccine. MMR, OPV, BCG = live attenuated.

Q9. NEET PG 2024
Which fungal pathogen is dimorphic and seen in AIDS patients with multiple oral ulcers and hepatosplenomegaly?
◦ A. Candida albicans
◦ B. Cryptococcus neoformans
◦ C. Histoplasma capsulatum
◦ D. Aspergillus fumigatus
✅ Ans: C. Histoplasma capsulatum
Explanation: Seen in immunocompromised; intracellular yeast in macrophages.

Q10. NEET PG 2024
An HIV-positive patient develops cryptococcal meningitis. What is the best diagnostic test?
◦ A. CSF Gram stain
◦ B. India ink
◦ C. Latex agglutination for capsule antigen
◦ D. CSF culture
✅ Ans: C. Latex agglutination
Explanation: Detects capsular polysaccharide antigen – highly sensitive and specific.

Clinical recall + stain & media + hot infections from recent trends

---

Q11.
A patient presents with bloody diarrhea. Culture shows motile, lactose non-fermenting gram-negative bacilli. What is the most likely organism?
◦ A. Shigella
◦ B. Salmonella
◦ C. E. coli
◦ D. Klebsiella
✅ Ans: B. Salmonella
Explanation: Shigella = non-motile; Salmonella = motile, H_2S positive, NLF.

Q12.
Which bacterial toxin acts by ADP-ribosylation of EF-2?
◦ A. Cholera toxin
◦ B. Pertussis toxin
◦ C. Diphtheria toxin

◦ D. Botulinum toxin

✅ Ans: C. Diphtheria toxin

Explanation: Inhibits protein synthesis → cell death → pseudomembrane.

Q13.
Which virus has a segmented RNA genome?

◦ A. Influenza virus
◦ B. Measles virus
◦ C. Rabies virus
◦ D. Dengue virus

✅ Ans: A. Influenza virus

Explanation: Orthomyxovirus with 8 RNA segments → antigenic shift.

Q14.
Which test is used for diagnosis of HIV infection in neonates?

◦ A. ELISA
◦ B. Western blot
◦ C. HIV DNA PCR
◦ D. Rapid antibody test

✅ Ans: C. HIV DNA PCR

Explanation: Maternal antibodies interfere with ELISA; PCR detects proviral DNA.

Q15.
Which fungal pathogen is visualized by India ink stain?

◦ A. Candida
◦ B. Aspergillus
◦ C. Cryptococcus
◦ D. Mucor

✅ Ans: C. Cryptococcus

Explanation: India ink shows clear halo around yeast (capsule).

Q16. NEET PG 2021
Which medium is used for culture of Mycobacterium tuberculosis?

◦ A. Thayer-Martin
◦ B. Chocolate agar
◦ C. Löwenstein–Jensen medium
◦ D. MacConkey agar

✅ Ans: C. Löwenstein–Jensen medium

Explanation: Egg-based medium; colonies appear after 2–8 weeks.

Q17. NEET PG 2021
A young girl has foul-smelling green vaginal discharge. Wet mount shows motile trophozoites. Likely pathogen?

◦ A. Candida
◦ B. Gardnerella
◦ C. Trichomonas
◦ D. Neisseria

✅ Ans: C. Trichomonas

Explanation: Flagellated protozoa; causes strawberry cervix, diagnosed on saline wet mount.

Q18. NEET PG 2021
Which DNA virus replicates in cytoplasm?

◦ A. Hepatitis B
◦ B. Herpes
◦ C. Poxvirus
◦ D. Papillomavirus

✅ Ans: C. Poxvirus

Explanation: Exception to the rule; poxvirus carries its own DNA-dependent RNA polymerase.

Q19. NEET PG 2021
Which of the following is the most effective sterilization method for heat-sensitive surgical instruments?

◦ A. Autoclave
◦ B. Dry heat

◦ C. Ethylene oxide gas
◦ D. UV rays
✅ Ans: C. Ethylene oxide gas
Explanation: Used for plastic, heat-labile items. Alkylates DNA/RNA.

Q20. NEET PG 2021
Which antibody is detected in the Weil–Felix test?
◦ A. IgG
◦ B. IgA
◦ C. IgE
◦ D. Heterophile antibody
✅ Ans: D. Heterophile antibody
Explanation: Cross-reacts with Proteus OX strains in rickettsial infections.

🎯 Focus: Gram stains, parasitology, virology, and repeat topics

---

📕 NEET PG Microbiology PYQs – Q21 to Q30 (2020–2019)

Q21. NEET PG 2020
Which gram-negative diplococcus grows on chocolate agar and ferments glucose only?
◦ A. Neisseria gonorrhoeae
◦ B. Neisseria meningitidis
◦ C. Moraxella catarrhalis
◦ D. Haemophilus influenzae
✅ Ans: A. Neisseria gonorrhoeae
Explanation: Oxidase-positive, glucose fermenter; grows on Thayer–Martin or chocolate agar.

Q22. NEET PG 2020
Charcot–Leyden crystals in stool are diagnostic of:
◦ A. Hookworm
◦ B. Ascaris
◦ C. E. histolytica
◦ D. Eosinophilic enteritis
✅ Ans: D. Eosinophilic enteritis
Explanation: Crystals formed from eosinóphil breakdown; seen in allergic or parasitic GI disease.

Q23. NEET PG 2020
Which of the following viruses is oncogenic?
◦ A. Coxsackievirus
◦ B. Rotavirus
◦ C. Epstein–Barr virus
◦ D. Rhinovirus
✅ Ans: C. Epstein–Barr virus
Explanation: Associated with nasopharyngeal carcinoma, Burkitt lymphoma.

Q24. NEET PG 2020
Hepatitis B surface antigen (HBsAg) is first detectable in:
◦ A. Blood
◦ B. Urine
◦ C. CSF
◦ D. Saliva
✅ Ans: A. Blood
Explanation: HBsAg is the earliest marker of infection and appears in blood 1–10 weeks post-exposure.

Q25. NEET PG 2020
A patient presents with hydatid cyst in liver. Which test is most specific?
◦ A. ELISA
◦ B. Indirect hemagglutination
◦ C. Casoni test
◦ D. Arc 5 precipitation
✅ Ans: D. Arc 5 precipitation
Explanation: Highly specific

immunodiffusion test for Echinococcus granulosus.

Q26. NEET PG 2019
Which of the following bacteria is catalase positive?
◦ A. Streptococcus
◦ B. Staphylococcus
◦ C. Enterococcus
◦ D. Lactobacillus
✅ Ans: B. Staphylococcus
Explanation: Catalase test differentiates Staph (+) from Strep (−).

Q27. NEET PG 2019
Which of the following is used to detect latent tuberculosis infection?
◦ A. BACTEC culture
◦ B. Ziehl–Neelsen stain
◦ C. GeneXpert
◦ D. Interferon gamma release assay (IGRA)
✅ Ans: D. IGRA
Explanation: Measures T-cell release of IFN-γ in response to TB antigens. No cross-reactivity with BCG.

Q28. NEET PG 2019
Which virus is transmitted through a segmented RNA genome and is capable of antigenic shift?
◦ A. Rotavirus
◦ B. Dengue virus
◦ C. HIV
◦ D. Hepatitis C
✅ Ans: A. Rotavirus
Explanation: Belongs to Reoviridae family; has 11 segments → antigenic shift.

Q29. NEET PG 2019
A man working with sheep develops a painless black necrotic eschar. Organism?
◦ A. Yersinia pestis
◦ B. Bacillus anthracis
◦ C. Clostridium perfringens
◦ D. Mycobacterium ulcerans
✅ Ans: B. Bacillus anthracis
Explanation: Cutaneous anthrax – classic painless black eschar.

Q30. NEET PG 2019
An HIV patient presents with chronic diarrhea. Modified acid-fast stain reveals oval acid-fast oocysts. Likely pathogen?
◦ A. Cryptosporidium
◦ B. Cyclospora
◦ C. Giardia
◦ D. Isospora
✅ Ans: A. Cryptosporidium
Explanation: Acid-fast oocysts in stool; chronic diarrhea in immunocompromised.

🎯 Focus: Cultures, spores, viral infections, high-yield clinical sets

---

Q31. NEET PG 2018
Culture medium for Vibrio cholerae?
◦ A. TCBS
◦ B. MacConkey
◦ C. Blood agar
◦ D. Loeffler's medium
✅ Ans: A. TCBS
Explanation: Thiosulfate–Citrate–Bile Salts–Sucrose medium; V. cholerae produces yellow colonies.

Q32. NEET PG 2018

A 5-year-old presents with sore throat and bull neck appearance. Culture shows gram-positive rods with club-shaped ends. Organism?
◦ A. Corynebacterium diphtheriae
◦ B. Haemophilus influenzae
◦ C. Streptococcus pyogenes
◦ D. Mycobacterium tuberculosis
✅ Ans: A. Corynebacterium diphtheriae
Explanation: Gram-positive bacilli with metachromatic granules, causing pseudomembrane and "bull neck".

Q33. NEET PG 2018
A child presents with rash and Koplik spots. Diagnosis?
◦ A. Rubella
◦ B. Measles
◦ C. Scarlet fever
◦ D. Chickenpox
✅ Ans: B. Measles
Explanation: Koplik spots (bluish-white spots opposite molars) precede the maculopapular rash.

Q34. NEET PG 2018
Which hepatitis virus is DNA-based and partially double-stranded?
◦ A. HAV
◦ B. HBV
◦ C. HCV
◦ D. HEV
✅ Ans: B. HBV
Explanation: Hepadnavirus family; reverse transcribes DNA → RNA → DNA.

Q35. NEET PG 2018
A patient bitten by a stray dog develops hydrophobia and photophobia. What will be seen in autopsy brain tissue?
◦ A. Cowdry bodies
◦ B. Negri bodies
◦ C. Owl eye inclusion
◦ D. Lewy bodies
✅ Ans: B. Negri bodies
Explanation: Seen in hippocampus and Purkinje cells in rabies.

Q36. NEET PG 2017
A 4-month-old child presents with pneumonia and staccato cough. Conjunctivitis is also noted. Likely organism?
◦ A. Chlamydia trachomatis
◦ B. RSV
◦ C. Streptococcus pneumoniae
◦ D. Haemophilus influenzae
✅ Ans: A. Chlamydia trachomatis
Explanation: Neonatal inclusion conjunctivitis + afebrile pneumonia with staccato cough.

Q37. NEET PG 2017
Tissue nematode diagnosed via muscle biopsy:
◦ A. Wuchereria bancrofti
◦ B. Loa loa
◦ C. Trichinella spiralis
◦ D. Onchocerca volvulus
✅ Ans: C. Trichinella spiralis
Explanation: Larvae encyst in striated muscle → myalgia, eosinophilia.

Q38. NEET PG 2017
Which is the most heat-resistant bacterial structure?
◦ A. Capsule
◦ B. Flagella
◦ C. Spores
◦ D. Pili
✅ Ans: C. Spores

Explanation: Spores (e.g., Bacillus, Clostridium) survive boiling, disinfectants, radiation.

Q39. NEET PG 2017
Gram-negative diplococci causing urethritis:
◦ A. Neisseria gonorrhoeae
◦ B. Chlamydia trachomatis
◦ C. Mycoplasma hominis
◦ D. Haemophilus ducreyi
✓ Ans: A. Neisseria gonorrhoeae
Explanation: Seen as intracellular gram-negative diplococci in PMNs on smear.

Q40. NEET PG 2017
Bacterial organism with swarming motility:
◦ A. E. coli
◦ B. Proteus mirabilis
◦ C. Klebsiella
◦ D. Salmonella
✓ Ans: B. Proteus mirabilis
Explanation: Rapid spreading growth on agar; urease positive, causes UTI with struvite stones.

Focus: Media, mycology, parasites, virology, and microbiological principles

---

Q41. NEET PG 2016
A 45-year-old farmer presents with a slowly progressing painless ulcer on the foot. KOH mount shows broad-based budding yeast. Diagnosis?
◦ A. Histoplasma
◦ B. Cryptococcus
◦ C. Blastomyces
◦ D. Aspergillus
✓ Ans: C. Blastomyces
Explanation: Broad-based budding, dimorphic fungus; endemic to Mississippi river valley.

Q42. NEET PG 2016
Which bacterial toxin increases intracellular cAMP?
◦ A. Shiga toxin
◦ B. Heat-stable toxin (E. coli)
◦ C. Cholera toxin
◦ D. Diphtheria toxin
✓ Ans: C. Cholera toxin
Explanation: ADP-ribosylates Gs → ↑ adenylate cyclase → ↑ cAMP → watery diarrhea.

Q43. NEET PG 2016
Which of the following does NOT produce spores?
◦ A. Clostridium
◦ B. Bacillus
◦ C. Corynebacterium
◦ D. None of the above
✓ Ans: C. Corynebacterium
Explanation: Corynebacterium is non-spore forming; unlike Bacillus and Clostridium.

Q44. NEET PG 2015
Patient develops a painless ulcer on the external genitalia followed by multiple draining inguinal lymph nodes. Likely diagnosis?
◦ A. Chancroid
◦ B. LGV
◦ C. Syphilis
◦ D. Donovanosis
✓ Ans: B. Lymphogranuloma venereum (LGV)
Explanation: Caused by C. trachomatis L1–L3 → ulcer + buboes.

Q45. NEET PG 2015
Which of the following parasites causes anemia due to chronic blood loss?
◦ A. Ascaris
◦ B. Hookworm
◦ C. Trichuris
◦ D. Strongyloides
✅ Ans: B. Hookworm
Explanation: Hookworm (Ancylostoma/Necator) attaches to intestinal mucosa → chronic iron deficiency anemia.

Q46. NEET PG 2015
Which fungal infection shows "spherules filled with endospores"?
◦ A. Histoplasma
◦ B. Coccidioides
◦ C. Blastomyces
◦ D. Cryptococcus
✅ Ans: B. Coccidioides
Explanation: Dimorphic fungus; Coccidioides immitis = spherules with endospores in tissue.

Q47. NEET PG 2014
A patient presents with fever, cough, and hemoptysis. Sputum shows septate hyphae branching at acute angles. Most probable organism?
◦ A. Candida
◦ B. Mucor
◦ C. Aspergillus
◦ D. Histoplasma
✅ Ans: C. Aspergillus
Explanation: Acute angle branching, septate hyphae = hallmark of Aspergillus.

Q48. NEET PG 2014
Bacterial capsule helps in:
◦ A. Motility
◦ B. Sporulation
◦ C. Adherence
◦ D. Antiphagocytosis
✅ Ans: D. Antiphagocytosis
Explanation: Capsules prevent phagocytosis (e.g., S. pneumoniae, H. influenzae type B, N. meningitidis).

Q49. NEET PG 2014
Which virus shows "owl's eye" inclusions?
◦ A. EBV
◦ B. HSV
◦ C. CMV
◦ D. VZV
✅ Ans: C. CMV
Explanation: Large basophilic intranuclear inclusion seen in infected endothelial cells.

Q50. NEET PG 2014
A child develops fever, rash, and vesicles in the mouth and extremities. Most likely virus?
◦ A. Coxsackie A
◦ B. EBV
◦ C. VZV
◦ D. HSV-1
✅ Ans: A. Coxsackie A
Explanation: Classic presentation of hand-foot-and-mouth disease caused by Coxsackie A16.

Q51. A neonate with delayed separation of umbilical cord and recurrent infections has normal WBC count but absent pus formation. Likely defect?
◦ A. Chediak–Higashi syndrome

◦ B. Chronic granulomatous disease
◦ C. Leukocyte adhesion deficiency (LAD)
◦ D. SCID

✅ Ans: C. Leukocyte adhesion deficiency (LAD)

Explanation: Defective CD18 integrin → neutrophils can't exit circulation → no pus, high WBC.

Q52. Which bacteria produces sulfur granules in discharging sinus from jaw?
◦ A. Nocardia
◦ B. Actinomyces israelii
◦ C. Mycobacterium tuberculosis
◦ D. Clostridium perfringens

✅ Ans: B. Actinomyces israelii

Explanation: Gram-positive filamentous anaerobe. Yellow "sulfur granules" in cervicofacial actinomycosis.

Q53. A female with malodorous vaginal discharge has clue cells on wet mount. Most likely organism?
◦ A. Trichomonas vaginalis
◦ B. Gardnerella vaginalis
◦ C. Neisseria gonorrhoeae
◦ D. Candida albicans

✅ Ans: B. Gardnerella vaginalis

Explanation: Clue cells = epithelial cells covered with bacteria; fishy odor with KOH.

Q54. Which stain is used for Mycobacterium leprae in tissue biopsy?
◦ A. Ziehl–Neelsen
◦ B. Fite–Faraco
◦ C. PAS
◦ D. India ink

✅ Ans: B. Fite–Faraco

Explanation: Modified acid-fast stain used for visualizing M. leprae in skin lesions.

Q55. A child presents with perianal itching at night. Transparent adhesive tape is used to detect eggs. Which parasite?
◦ A. Ascaris
◦ B. Enterobius vermicularis
◦ C. Trichuris
◦ D. Strongyloides

✅ Ans: B. Enterobius vermicularis

Explanation: Pinworm eggs seen on tape test; classic for nocturnal itching.

Q56. Which test is used for diagnosis of syphilis during early primary stage?
◦ A. VDRL
◦ B. TPHA
◦ C. Dark-field microscopy
◦ D. FTA-ABS

✅ Ans: C. Dark-field microscopy

Explanation: Direct visualization of motile Treponema from chancre fluid.

Q57. In case of malaria with ring forms and banana-shaped gametocytes, which species is most likely?
◦ A. P. vivax
◦ B. P. falciparum
◦ C. P. malariae
◦ D. P. ovale

✅ Ans: B. P. falciparum

Explanation: Ring forms in RBCs and crescent-shaped gametocytes are pathognomonic.

Q58. Which organism causes multiple vesicular skin lesions and is detected by Tzanck smear?
◦ A. HSV

◦ B. VZV
◦ C. Coxsackie
◦ D. Measles
✅ Ans: A. HSV
Explanation: HSV shows multinucleated giant cells with inclusion bodies on Tzanck smear.

Q59. A renal transplant patient on immunosuppressants develops hemorrhagic cystitis. Likely virus?
◦ A. BK virus
◦ B. CMV
◦ C. JC virus
◦ D. EBV
✅ Ans: A. BK virus
Explanation: Polyomavirus that causes hemorrhagic cystitis in renal transplant patients.

Q60. Which bacteria has a polysaccharide capsule and is bile soluble?
◦ A. Streptococcus pyogenes
◦ B. Streptococcus agalactiae
◦ C. Streptococcus pneumoniae
◦ D. Enterococcus faecalis
✅ Ans: C. Streptococcus pneumoniae
Explanation: Lancet-shaped diplococci; optochin-sensitive, bile soluble, capsulated.

Q61. Which DNA virus is enveloped and replicates in cytoplasm?
◦ A. Hepatitis B virus
◦ B. Adenovirus
◦ C. Herpes simplex virus
◦ D. Poxvirus
✅ Ans: D. Poxvirus
Explanation: Only DNA virus that replicates in cytoplasm using its own polymerases.

Q62. Which parasite shows lateral spine in ova and is associated with hematuria?
◦ A. Schistosoma mansoni
◦ B. Schistosoma japonicum
◦ C. Schistosoma haematobium
◦ D. Fasciola hepatica
✅ Ans: C. Schistosoma haematobium
Explanation: Found in venous plexus of bladder → terminal hematuria, squamous cell carcinoma risk.

Q63. Which fungal infection is most commonly associated with bird droppings and causes meningitis in AIDS patients?
◦ A. Histoplasmosis
◦ B. Cryptococcosis
◦ C. Candidiasis
◦ D. Aspergillosis
✅ Ans: B. Cryptococcosis
Explanation: Capsulated yeast, India ink test, latex agglutination for antigen detection.

Q64. Which of the following acts via ADP-ribosylation of G-protein to increase cAMP?
◦ A. Botulinum toxin
◦ B. Cholera toxin
◦ C. Tetanus toxin
◦ D. Shiga toxin
✅ Ans: B. Cholera toxin
Explanation: Activates Gs → ↑ adenylate cyclase → ↑ cAMP → secretory diarrhea.

Q65. A case of lymphatic filariasis with nocturnal periodicity. Which is the best

test?
◦ A. Blood smear at 6 pm
◦ B. Blood smear at noon
◦ C. Blood smear at 2 am
◦ D. Blood smear at 10 am

✅ Ans: C. Blood smear at 2 am
Explanation: W. bancrofti shows nocturnal periodicity – best seen in peripheral smear at midnight.

Q66. A patient develops pneumonia after bird exposure. Gram stain negative. Which organism?
◦ A. Histoplasma
◦ B. Chlamydophila psittaci
◦ C. Cryptococcus
◦ D. Coxiella

✅ Ans: B. Chlamydophila psittaci
Explanation: Zoonotic atypical pneumonia; psittacosis → seen in bird handlers.

Q67. Which bacterial structure is responsible for adherence to uroepithelial cells?
◦ A. Flagella
◦ B. Capsule
◦ C. Fimbriae (pili)
◦ D. Spores

✅ Ans: C. Fimbriae (pili)
Explanation: Type 1 and P fimbriae mediate adhesion to urinary tract epithelium in E. coli UTI.

Q68. An AIDS patient presents with white oral patches that are easily scraped off. KOH mount shows pseudohyphae. Likely pathogen?
◦ A. Aspergillus
◦ B. Candida albicans
◦ C. Cryptococcus
◦ D. Histoplasma

✅ Ans: B. Candida albicans
Explanation: Pseudohyphae with budding yeast; scrapable oral thrush in immunosuppressed patients.

Q69. Which of the following is a slow virus disease?
◦ A. HSV
◦ B. PML (JC virus)
◦ C. Rabies
◦ D. Measles

✅ Ans: B. PML (Progressive multifocal leukoencephalopathy)
Explanation: JC virus in immunocompromised → demyelination of CNS → slow viral CNS disease.

Q70. An infection shows sulfur granules, is anaerobic, and produces branching filaments. Which one?
◦ A. Nocardia
◦ B. Actinomyces
◦ C. Clostridium
◦ D. Bacillus

✅ Ans: B. Actinomyces
Explanation: Anaerobic, gram-positive filamentous bacteria → cervicofacial actinomycosis.

🎯 Focus: Bloodborne viruses, toxins, vaccine types, lab techniques, and differentiators

---

Q71. Which hepatitis virus is associated with maximum chronicity and liver cancer risk?
◦ A. HAV
◦ B. HBV
◦ C. HCV
◦ D. HEV

✅ Ans: C. HCV
Explanation: RNA virus, high mutation rate, no proofreading → chronicity + hepatocellular carcinoma.

Q72. A patient develops pseudomembranous colitis after clindamycin therapy. Which toxin is implicated?
◦ A. Exotoxin A of C. difficile
◦ B. Endotoxin of E. coli
◦ C. Enterotoxin of B. cereus
◦ D. Heat-labile toxin of ETEC
✅ Ans: A. Exotoxin A of C. difficile
Explanation: Toxin A (enterotoxin) → inflammation; Toxin B (cytotoxin) → mucosal damage.

Q73. Which vaccine is contraindicated in pregnancy?
◦ A. Hepatitis B
◦ B. Influenza (inactivated)
◦ C. Rubella (MMR)
◦ D. Tdap
✅ Ans: C. Rubella (MMR)
Explanation: Live vaccines are contraindicated in pregnancy due to fetal teratogenic risk.

Q74. Which immunoglobulin crosses the placenta?
◦ A. IgA
◦ B. IgM
◦ C. IgG
◦ D. IgE
✅ Ans: C. IgG
Explanation: Only IgG crosses placenta → provides passive immunity to neonates.

Q75. An AIDS patient presents with multiple non-painful skin nodules. Biopsy shows vascular proliferation with slit-like spaces. Likely cause?
◦ A. CMV
◦ B. EBV
◦ C. HHV-8
◦ D. HPV
✅ Ans: C. HHV-8
Explanation: Kaposi sarcoma – vascular tumor caused by Human Herpesvirus-8.

Q76. Which virus causes congenital sensorineural hearing loss and periventricular calcifications?
◦ A. HSV-2
◦ B. CMV
◦ C. Rubella
◦ D. Toxoplasma
✅ Ans: B. CMV
Explanation: Most common congenital viral infection; causes microcephaly, chorioretinitis.

Q77. Which of the following organisms is urease positive and causes struvite stones?
◦ A. Proteus
◦ B. E. coli
◦ C. Pseudomonas
◦ D. Klebsiella
✅ Ans: A. Proteus
Explanation: Urease → ↑ pH → precipitation of magnesium ammonium phosphate (struvite) stones.

Q78. Which test is used to diagnose bacterial meningitis and assess antibiotic susceptibility?
◦ A. CSF Gram stain
◦ B. Latex agglutination

◦ C. Culture & sensitivity
◦ D. India ink
✅ Ans: C. Culture & sensitivity
Explanation: Gold standard for diagnosis + antibiotic selection.

Q79. A case of post-burn wound infection grows blue-green pigment on agar. Likely pathogen?
◦ A. S. aureus
◦ B. Klebsiella
◦ C. Pseudomonas
◦ D. Proteus
✅ Ans: C. Pseudomonas
Explanation: Produces pyocyanin and pyoverdin → greenish pigment; oxidase positive.

Q80. Which of the following is a DNA virus?
◦ A. Dengue
◦ B. Rabies
◦ C. Hepatitis B
◦ D. Measles
✅ Ans: C. Hepatitis B
Explanation: HBV = Hepadnavirus, partially double-stranded DNA with reverse transcriptase.

🎯 Focus: TB diagnostics, leprosy, Gram-positives, and infectious disease pearls

---

Q81. Which test is used to detect rifampicin resistance in TB?
◦ A. Mantoux test
◦ B. BACTEC
◦ C. GeneXpert (CBNAAT)
◦ D. Ziehl–Neelsen stain
✅ Ans: C. GeneXpert
Explanation: Detects M. tuberculosis DNA and rifampicin resistance via rpoB gene mutations.

Q82. Lepromin test is:
◦ A. Diagnostic test
◦ B. Test of cell-mediated immunity
◦ C. Serological test
◦ D. Test for antibody response
✅ Ans: B. Test of cell-mediated immunity
Explanation: Positive in tuberculoid leprosy; negative in lepromatous leprosy.

Q83. Which Gram-positive cocci shows bile solubility and optochin sensitivity?
◦ A. Staphylococcus aureus
◦ B. Streptococcus pneumoniae
◦ C. Enterococcus faecalis
◦ D. Streptococcus viridans
✅ Ans: B. Streptococcus pneumoniae
Explanation: Lancet-shaped diplococci, alpha-hemolytic, optochin-sensitive, bile soluble.

Q84. Which pathogen causes genital ulcer + painful lymphadenopathy (buboes)?
◦ A. Treponema pallidum
◦ B. Haemophilus ducreyi
◦ C. Chlamydia trachomatis
◦ D. Klebsiella granulomatis
✅ Ans: B. Haemophilus ducreyi
Explanation: Chancroid → painful, ragged ulcer + tender lymphadenopathy ("school of fish" on smear).

Q85. Which one is not a dimorphic fungus?
◦ A. Histoplasma

◦ B. Candida
◦ C. Sporothrix
◦ D. Blastomyces
✅ Ans: B. Candida
Explanation: Candida is yeast with pseudohyphae; not a true dimorphic fungus like the others.

Q86. Which test is used to detect presence of capsulated yeast in CSF?
◦ A. Ziehl–Neelsen stain
◦ B. KOH mount
◦ C. Latex agglutination
◦ D. Tzanck smear
✅ Ans: C. Latex agglutination
Explanation: For Cryptococcus neoformans, detects capsular antigen in CSF.

Q87. Which of the following causes flaccid paralysis?
◦ A. Tetanus
◦ B. Botulism
◦ C. Rabies
◦ D. Poliovirus
✅ Ans: B. Botulism
Explanation: Botulinum toxin inhibits ACh release → flaccid paralysis.

Q88. Which bacterium is associated with cold agglutinin hemolytic anemia?
◦ A. Mycoplasma pneumoniae
◦ B. Legionella
◦ C. Chlamydia
◦ D. Bordetella
✅ Ans: A. Mycoplasma pneumoniae
Explanation: Causes atypical pneumonia and produces IgM that cross-reacts with RBCs.

Q89. Which virus uses reverse transcriptase enzyme for replication?
◦ A. HCV
◦ B. HBV
◦ C. Influenza
◦ D. Measles
✅ Ans: B. HBV
Explanation: HBV is a DNA virus that replicates via reverse transcription.

Q90. Which test is used to detect latent TB infection especially in BCG-vaccinated individuals?
◦ A. Mantoux test
◦ B. Interferon-gamma release assay (IGRA)
◦ C. GeneXpert
◦ D. Ziehl–Neelsen stain
✅ Ans: B. IGRA
Explanation: No cross-reactivity with BCG; detects T-cell release of IFN-γ in response to TB antigens.

Q91. A 30-year-old with exposure to unpasteurized milk develops undulant fever and hepatosplenomegaly. Organism?
◦ A. Leptospira
◦ B. Brucella
◦ C. Salmonella
◦ D. Coxiella
✅ Ans: B. Brucella
Explanation: Zoonotic infection, undulating fever; culture on Castaneda medium or blood culture.

Q92.
Which vaccine contains live attenuated virus?
◦ A. Hepatitis B

◦ B. Rabies (IM)
◦ C. Measles
◦ D. IPV (Inactivated Polio Vaccine)

✅ Ans: C. Measles

Explanation: MMR is a live attenuated vaccine. Hep B = recombinant, IPV = killed.

Q93. Which bacterial structure determines serotype classification in E. coli (e.g., O157:H7)?

◦ A. Capsule
◦ B. Flagella
◦ C. Lipopolysaccharide (O antigen)
◦ D. Pili

✅ Ans: C. Lipopolysaccharide (O antigen)

Explanation: O antigen = outer LPS; H = flagella, K = capsule.

Q94. A 5-year-old with sore throat later develops facial puffiness and hematuria. Which strain is implicated?

◦ A. Streptococcus agalactiae
◦ B. Streptococcus pyogenes
◦ C. Staphylococcus aureus
◦ D. Enterococcus faecalis

✅ Ans: B. Streptococcus pyogenes

Explanation: Post-streptococcal glomerulonephritis follows nephritogenic strains of group A beta-hemolytic strep.

Q95. A 10-year-old presents with sandpaper rash, strawberry tongue, and fever. Likely organism?

◦ A. Staphylococcus aureus
◦ B. Streptococcus pyogenes
◦ C. Corynebacterium diphtheriae
◦ D. Neisseria meningitidis

✅ Ans: B. Streptococcus pyogenes

Explanation: Scarlet fever; due to erythrogenic exotoxin of S. pyogenes.

Q96. A pathogen shows tumbling motility and is intracellular. Causes abortion in pregnant women. Likely organism?

◦ A. Listeria monocytogenes
◦ B. Toxoplasma gondii
◦ C. CMV
◦ D. Rubella

✅ Ans: A. Listeria monocytogenes

Explanation: Gram-positive rod with actin rocket tails, survives inside macrophages.

Q97. Which parasite causes chorioretinitis, hydrocephalus, and intracranial calcification in neonates?

◦ A. Toxoplasma gondii
◦ B. Rubella
◦ C. CMV
◦ D. HSV

✅ Ans: A. Toxoplasma gondii

Explanation: Congenital toxoplasmosis triad = hydrocephalus, chorioretinitis, calcifications.

Q98.
A virus with bullet-shaped morphology:

◦ A. Rabies
◦ B. Dengue
◦ C. Rotavirus
◦ D. Influenza

✅ Ans: A. Rabies

Explanation: Rhabdovirus family; bullet-shaped virions seen on EM.

Q99. Which antibody provides mucosal immunity?

◦ A. IgG

◦ B. IgE
◦ C. IgA
◦ D. IgM

✅ Ans: C. IgA

Explanation: Secretory IgA protects mucosa (gut, respiratory, urogenital).

Q100.

Which bacteria forms spores and causes severe watery diarrhea and abdominal cramps after meat consumption?

◦ A. Clostridium perfringens
◦ B. Bacillus cereus
◦ C. Shigella
◦ D. Vibrio cholerae

✅ Ans: A. Clostridium perfringens

Explanation: Heat-labile enterotoxin from ingested spores → late-onset food poisoning.

Revision Boost: 50 Bonus Microbiology PYQs

Q1. A child with pharyngitis develops facial edema and cola-colored urine. Urinalysis shows RBC casts. Likely causative organism?

◦ A. Streptococcus pyogenes
◦ B. Staphylococcus aureus
◦ C. Neisseria meningitidis
◦ D. Enterococcus

✅ Ans: A. Streptococcus pyogenes

Explanation: Classic post-streptococcal glomerulonephritis → nephritogenic strains of GAS.

Q2. Which pathogen causes descending flaccid paralysis?

◦ A. Tetanus
◦ B. Rabies
◦ C. Botulinum toxin
◦ D. Poliovirus

✅ Ans: C. Botulinum toxin

Explanation: Inhibits ACh release → symmetric descending weakness → floppy baby.

Q3. Which virus shows owl's eye intranuclear inclusions?

◦ A. HSV
◦ B. EBV
◦ C. CMV
◦ D. HPV

✅ Ans: C. CMV

Explanation: Seen in endothelial cells, most common congenital viral infection.

Q4. A case of lumpy jaw in a farmer shows sulfur granules. What's the likely organism?

◦ A. Actinomyces israelii
◦ B. Nocardia asteroides
◦ C. Clostridium tetani
◦ D. Bacillus anthracis

✅ Ans: A. Actinomyces israelii

Explanation: Anaerobic gram-positive filamentous bacilli; part of normal oral flora.

Q5. Which parasite causes autoinfection and can persist in immunocompromised hosts?

◦ A. Strongyloides stercoralis
◦ B. Ancylostoma
◦ C. Trichuris
◦ D. Taenia solium

✅ Ans: A. Strongyloides stercoralis

Explanation: Penetrates intact skin → autoinfection → hyperinfection in immunocompromised.

Q6. India ink test is diagnostic for:

◦ A. Candida
◦ B. Cryptococcus
◦ C. Aspergillus
◦ D. Histoplasma

✅ Ans: B. Cryptococcus

Explanation: Shows clear halo due to polysaccharide capsule.

Q7. Which toxin inhibits glycine and GABA release?

◦ A. Botulinum
◦ B. Shiga

◦ C. Tetanospasmin
◦ D. Diphtheria

✅ Ans: C. Tetanospasmin

Explanation: Retrograde axonal transport → blocks inhibitory neurons → spastic paralysis.

Q8. Bacteria with swarming motility and urease positivity:

◦ A. E. coli
◦ B. Klebsiella
◦ C. Proteus mirabilis
◦ D. Pseudomonas

✅ Ans: C. Proteus mirabilis

Explanation: Swarming colonies; produces struvite stones.

Q9. Which bacterium lacks a peptidoglycan cell wall and is resistant to beta-lactams?

◦ A. Mycoplasma pneumoniae
◦ B. Mycobacterium tuberculosis
◦ C. Chlamydia
◦ D. Nocardia

✅ Ans: A. Mycoplasma pneumoniae

Explanation: Cell membrane contains sterols instead of cell wall.

Q10. What type of vaccine is BCG?

◦ A. Killed
◦ B. Live attenuated
◦ C. Subunit
◦ D. Recombinant protein

✅ Ans: B. Live attenuated

Explanation: Derived from Mycobacterium bovis; induces cell-mediated immunity.

Q11. Which of the following is a catalase-positive Gram-positive cocci in clusters?

◦ A. Streptococcus pyogenes
◦ B. Staphylococcus aureus
◦ C. Enterococcus
◦ D. Streptococcus pneumoniae

✅ Ans: B. Staphylococcus aureus

Explanation: Catalase and coagulase positive; produces golden-yellow colonies.

Q12. What is the vector of Lyme disease?

◦ A. Sandfly
◦ B. Ixodes tick
◦ C. Louse
◦ D. Flea

✅ Ans: B. Ixodes tick

Explanation: Transmits Borrelia burgdorferi; associated with deer and rodents.

Q13.Which viral infection is most associated with SSPE (Subacute sclerosing panencephalitis)?

◦ A. Rubella
◦ B. Measles
◦ C. Mumps
◦ D. CMV

✅ Ans: B. Measles

Explanation: Defective measles virus persists in CNS → slow progressive neurological degeneration.

Q14. A dimorphic fungus causing rose gardener's disease:

◦ A. Cryptococcus
◦ B. Sporothrix schenckii
◦ C. Histoplasma
◦ D. Candida

✅ Ans: B. Sporothrix schenckii

Explanation: Causes sporotrichosis; lymphocutaneous nodules in chain.

Q15. Which test is used to screen for HIV in blood banks?
◦ A. Western blot
◦ B. ELISA
◦ C. PCR
◦ D. VDRL

✅ Ans: B. ELISA
Explanation: Highly sensitive, used for mass screening. Western blot/PCR for confirmation.

Q16. Which parasite causes hematuria and bladder wall granulomas?
◦ A. Schistosoma haematobium
◦ B. S. mansoni
◦ C. Fasciola hepatica
◦ D. Trichinella

✅ Ans: A. Schistosoma haematobium
Explanation: Associated with squamous cell carcinoma of the bladder.

Q17. Antibody associated with mucosal surfaces:
◦ A. IgM
◦ B. IgG
◦ C. IgA
◦ D. IgE

✅ Ans: C. IgA
Explanation: Found in secretions (tears, saliva, GI, milk); protects mucosal surfaces.

Q18. Which organism causes pneumonia with hyponatremia?
◦ A. Legionella pneumophila
◦ B. Mycoplasma pneumoniae
◦ C. Streptococcus pneumoniae
◦ D. H. influenzae

✅ Ans: A. Legionella pneumophila
Explanation: Atypical pneumonia + CNS/GI symptoms + low Na^+; culture on BCYE agar.

Q19. Which virus is non-enveloped and causes conjunctivitis outbreaks (shipyard eye)?
◦ A. HSV
◦ B. Adenovirus
◦ C. CMV
◦ D. Measles

✅ Ans: B. Adenovirus
Explanation: Serotype 8, 19, 37 → epidemic keratoconjunctivitis; spreads via fomites.

Q20. A bacterial capsule is best demonstrated by:
◦ A. Gram stain
◦ B. Ziehl–Neelsen
◦ C. India ink
◦ D. Negative stain

✅ Ans: D. Negative stain
Explanation: Background stains; capsule appears as halo (e.g., Cryptococcus, Klebsiella).

Q21. A patient with sinusitis, fever, and black necrotic nasal tissue. Likely pathogen?
◦ A. Aspergillus
◦ B. Mucor
◦ C. Cryptococcus
◦ D. Candida

✅ Ans: B. Mucor
Explanation: Angioinvasive, especially in diabetics → black eschar in nasal cavity (mucormycosis).

Q22. A gardener has multiple non-healing ulcers along lymphatics. Culture grows cigar-shaped yeast. Likely

pathogen?
◦ A. Histoplasma
◦ B. Sporothrix schenckii
◦ C. Candida
◦ D. Cryptococcus

✅ Ans: B. Sporothrix schenckii
Explanation: Dimorphic, rose handler's disease → nodular lymphangitis.

Q23. A 2-month-old infant presents with coughing spells followed by vomiting. CBC shows lymphocytosis. Most likely organism?
◦ A. RSV
◦ B. Bordetella pertussis
◦ C. Adenovirus
◦ D. Parainfluenza

✅ Ans: B. Bordetella pertussis
Explanation: Whooping cough; lymphocytosis due to pertussis toxin.

Q24. A woman with greenish vaginal discharge and motile flagellates on saline mount. Diagnosis?
◦ A. Bacterial vaginosis
◦ B. Trichomoniasis
◦ C. Candidiasis
◦ D. Gonorrhea

✅ Ans: B. Trichomoniasis
Explanation: Trichomonas vaginalis – flagellated protozoa seen on wet mount.

Q25. Which organism has "safety-pin" bipolar staining?
◦ A. Yersinia pestis
◦ B. Haemophilus ducreyi
◦ C. Francisella
◦ D. Pasteurella

✅ Ans: A. Yersinia pestis
Explanation: Bipolar staining with Wayson or Giemsa stain; plague bacillus.

Q26. Test used to identify Clostridium difficile toxin:
◦ A. Culture
◦ B. Gram stain
◦ C. ELISA
◦ D. Schaeffer–Fulton

✅ Ans: C. ELISA
Explanation: Detects Toxin A and/or B in stool.

Q27. Which virus has segmented RNA and is capable of reassortment?
◦ A. Influenza
◦ B. Measles
◦ C. Rabies
◦ D. Dengue

✅ Ans: A. Influenza
Explanation: Orthomyxovirus, 8 segments → antigenic shift (pandemics).

Q28. A 25-year-old man presents with painless genital ulcer and painless lymphadenopathy. Most likely cause?
◦ A. Haemophilus ducreyi
◦ B. Treponema pallidum
◦ C. Chlamydia trachomatis
◦ D. Klebsiella granulomatis

✅ Ans: B. Treponema pallidum
Explanation: Primary syphilis; dark-field microscopy for diagnosis.

Q29. Which parasite is acid-fast positive in stool and causes severe diarrhea in HIV patients?
◦ A. Entamoeba
◦ B. Cryptosporidium
◦ C. Giardia
◦ D. Trichuris

✅ Ans: B. Cryptosporidium
Explanation: Oocysts seen with modified acid-fast stain; waterborne spread.

Q30. A non-motile, lactose non-fermenter bacillus causing bloody diarrhea in children:
◦ A. Shigella
◦ B. Salmonella
◦ C. EHEC
◦ D. Vibrio

✅ Ans: A. Shigella
Explanation: Non-motile, gram-negative bacillus → dysentery; shiga toxin may cause HUS.

Q31. Which of the following organisms is coagulase-positive?
◦ A. Streptococcus pyogenes
◦ B. Staphylococcus aureus
◦ C. Streptococcus pneumoniae
◦ D. Enterococcus faecalis

✅ Ans: B. Staphylococcus aureus
Explanation: Coagulase distinguishes S. aureus from other staph species.

Q32. Which immunoglobulin is responsible for anaphylaxis and parasitic immunity?
◦ A. IgA
◦ B. IgE
◦ C. IgG
◦ D. IgM

✅ Ans: B. IgE
Explanation: IgE binds mast cells/basophils → type I hypersensitivity.

Q33. Which bacteria shows double zone of hemolysis?
◦ A. Clostridium perfringens
◦ B. Streptococcus pyogenes
◦ C. E. coli
◦ D. Listeria monocytogenes

✅ Ans: A. Clostridium perfringens
Explanation: Inner beta + outer alpha hemolysis on blood agar.

Q34. Which mycobacterium is photochromogenic?
◦ A. M. kansasii
◦ B. M. tuberculosis
◦ C. M. avium
◦ D. M. leprae

✅ Ans: A. M. kansasii
Explanation: Scotochromogen = pigment in dark; Photochromogen = pigment in light.

Q35. Atypical lymphocytes seen in peripheral smear in:
◦ A. EBV infection
◦ B. CMV
◦ C. HIV
◦ D. HSV

✅ Ans: A. EBV
Explanation: Downey cells = reactive CD8+ T cells in infectious mononucleosis.

Q36. Pathogen causing pneumonia in alcoholics with red currant jelly sputum:
◦ A. Streptococcus pneumoniae
◦ B. Haemophilus influenzae
◦ C. Klebsiella pneumoniae
◦ D. Pseudomonas aeruginosa

✅ Ans: C. Klebsiella pneumoniae
Explanation: Gram-negative, encapsulated rod; mucoid colonies.

Q37. A pregnant woman exposed to cat litter develops chorioretinitis in newborn. Likely organism?
◦ A. Rubella
◦ B. Toxoplasma gondii
◦ C. CMV
◦ D. HSV
✅ Ans: B. Toxoplasma gondii
Explanation: Classic congenital toxoplasmosis — eye, brain, calcifications.

Q38. Antigenic drift in influenza is due to:
◦ A. Reassortment
◦ B. Mutation
◦ C. Conjugation
◦ D. Transformation
✅ Ans: B. Mutation
Explanation: Drift = point mutations → epidemics; shift = reassortment → pandemics.

Q39. Which bacteria is PYR positive and bacitracin sensitive?
◦ A. Streptococcus agalactiae
◦ B. Streptococcus pyogenes
◦ C. Enterococcus
◦ D. Viridans streptococci
✅ Ans: B. Streptococcus pyogenes
Explanation: Group A strep = bacitracin sensitive, PYR positive.

Q40.
Which parasite causes perianal itching in children?
◦ A. Ascaris
◦ B. Enterobius
◦ C. Trichuris
◦ D. Hookworm
✅ Ans: B. Enterobius
Explanation: Pinworm → diagnosed with Scotch tape test.

Q41. Which test detects TB antigen-specific interferon-gamma release?
◦ A. Mantoux
◦ B. GeneXpert
◦ C. IGRA
◦ D. Ziehl–Neelsen stain
✅ Ans: C. IGRA
Explanation: Interferon Gamma Release Assay detects latent TB, unaffected by BCG vaccine.

Q42. Which pathogen causes lockjaw with risus sardonicus?
◦ A. Clostridium tetani
◦ B. Clostridium botulinum
◦ C. Rabies
◦ D. Streptococcus pyogenes
✅ Ans: A. Clostridium tetani
Explanation: Tetanospasmin blocks GABA/glycine → spastic paralysis.

Q43. Which virus can integrate into host DNA and cause hepatocellular carcinoma?
◦ A. HCV
◦ B. HAV
◦ C. HEV
◦ D. HBV
✅ Ans: D. HBV
Explanation: HBV integrates into genome → chronic inflammation → malignancy.

Q44.
Which pathogen causes diarrhea and shows oocysts on modified acid-fast

stain?
◦ A. Giardia
◦ B. Entamoeba
◦ C. Cryptosporidium
◦ D. Trichuris
✅ Ans: C. Cryptosporidium
Explanation: Acid-fast oocysts in stool of immunocompromised patients.

Q45.
Vaccine containing purified capsular polysaccharide:
◦ A. OPV
◦ B. BCG
◦ C. Pneumococcal vaccine (PPSV23)
◦ D. MMR
✅ Ans: C. Pneumococcal vaccine (PPSV23)
Explanation: Capsular polysaccharide vaccine (T-cell independent).

Q46. Which virus is associated with Burkitt lymphoma?
◦ A. EBV
◦ B. CMV
◦ C. HHV-6
◦ D. HSV-1
✅ Ans: A. EBV
Explanation: Linked to Burkitt, nasopharyngeal carcinoma, Hodgkin's lymphoma.

Q47. A burn wound grows a grape-like smelling bacteria with blue-green pigment. Organism?
◦ A. Staphylococcus aureus
◦ B. Pseudomonas aeruginosa
◦ C. Streptococcus pyogenes
◦ D. Proteus
✅ Ans: B. Pseudomonas aeruginosa
Explanation: Produces pyocyanin, fruity odor; oxidase positive.

Q48.
Which parasite shows proglottids and scolex on stool microscopy?
◦ A. Giardia
◦ B. Hookworm
◦ C. Taenia
◦ D. Enterobius
✅ Ans: C. Taenia
Explanation: Tapeworm (Taenia solium/saginata); scolex has suckers ± hooks.

Q49. A patient with vesicular lesions on lips and gingiva. Tzanck smear shows multinucleated giant cells. Likely cause?
◦ A. HSV-1
◦ B. VZV
◦ C. Measles
◦ D. Coxsackie
✅ Ans: A. HSV-1
Explanation: Gingivostomatitis due to HSV; Tzanck = giant cells + Cowdry A inclusions.

Q50. Which virus is known for "steeple sign" on X-ray and barking cough?
◦ A. RSV
◦ B. Parainfluenza
◦ C. Adenovirus
◦ D. Influenza B
✅ Ans: B. Parainfluenza
Explanation: Causes croup; subglottic narrowing = steeple sign.

Microbiology – Bonus Add-On: 50 Rapidfire Recall Questions

1. Most common cause of food poisoning worldwide? → Campylobacter jejuni
2. DOC for typhoid fever? → Ceftriaxone
3. McCoy cell line used for? → Chlamydia
4. Vaccine for TB? → BCG (Live attenuated)
5. Spaghetti and meatballs appearance in stain? → Malassezia furfur
6. Acid-fast bacilli seen in? → Mycobacterium tuberculosis
7. Shape of Vibrio cholerae? → Comma shaped
8. India ink positive organism? → Cryptococcus neoformans
9. Dermatophytes affect? → Skin, hair, nails
10. Most common cause of UTI? → E. coli
11. Red pigment producing bacteria? → Serratia marcescens
12. Catalase positive fungi? → Aspergillus
13. Safety pin appearance on staining? → Yersinia pestis
14. Weil-Felix test used in? → Rickettsial infections
15. DOC for Pneumocystis jirovecii? → Trimethoprim-sulfamethoxazole
16. Non-motile protozoa? → Cryptosporidium
17. Swimmer's itch causative organism? → Schistosoma
18. Virus with reverse transcriptase? → HIV
19. Councilman bodies seen in? → Yellow fever (liver)
20. Downey cells seen in? → EBV infection (Infectious mononucleosis)
21. Owl's eye inclusion body? → CMV
22. TORCH infection with chorioretinitis? → Toxoplasmosis
23. DOC for amoebiasis? → Metronidazole
24. Most common cause of meningitis in neonates? → Group B Streptococcus
25. Leprosy bacillus discovered by? → G. H. Armauer Hansen
26. Cause of Montevideo fever? → Rickettsia typhi
27. Bacteria without cell wall? → Mycoplasma
28. HBsAg indicates? → Hepatitis B infection (active)
29. Councilman bodies found in? → Apoptotic hepatocytes (e.g., viral hepatitis)
30. Most sensitive test for TB? → PCR
31. Reverse transcriptase enzyme is seen in? → Retroviruses
32. Virus causing subacute sclerosing panencephalitis? → Measles virus
33. Most common agent for fungal meningitis in AIDS? → Cryptococcus neoformans
34. DOC for giardiasis? → Metronidazole
35. Which hepatitis virus is DNA? → Hepatitis B
36. Which parasite causes autoinfection? → Strongyloides stercoralis

37. Dog tapeworm causing hydatid cyst? → Echinococcus granulosus
38. Tzanck smear is used in? → Herpes simplex, Varicella-zoster
39. Cyst with four nuclei seen in? → Entamoeba histolytica
40. Trophozoites in stool in? → Amoebic dysentery
41. Lancefield classification is for? → Streptococci
42. DOC for MRSA? → Vancomycin
43. Spore-forming anaerobic gram-positive bacillus? → Clostridium
44. Schuffner's dots are seen in? → Plasmodium vivax
45. CSF finding in TB meningitis? → High protein, low sugar, lymphocytic
46. MC fungal infection in immunocompetent? → Dermatophytosis
47. Gram-negative diplococci in CSF? → Neisseria meningitidis
48. Blue green pus with fruity smell? → Pseudomonas aeruginosa
49. Oral thrush seen in? → Candida albicans
50. DOC for herpes zoster? → Acyclovir

Bacteria – Basic Classification & Examples

• Gram-positive cocci: Staphylococcus, Streptococcus
• Gram-positive rods: Bacillus, Clostridium, Corynebacterium
• Gram-negative cocci: Neisseria (gonorrhoeae, meningitidis)
• Gram-negative rods: E. coli, Salmonella, Shigella, Klebsiella
• Acid-fast bacteria: Mycobacterium tuberculosis, M. leprae
• Spirochetes: Treponema, Leptospira, Borrelia

Common Bacteria by Shape and Oxygen Requirement

Shape	Aerobic / Anaerobic	Examples
Cocci	Aerobic	Staphylococcus, Streptococcus
Cocci	Anaerobic	Peptostreptococcus
Rods	Aerobic	Bacillus, Listeria, Pseudomonas
Rods	Anaerobic	Clostridium, Bacteroides
Spiral	Microaerophilic	Helicobacter pylori

Bacterial Toxins – Quick Recall

• Corynebacterium diphtheriae – Exotoxin inhibits EF-2 → pseudomembrane
• Clostridium tetani – Tetanospasmin blocks GABA & glycine → spastic paralysis
• Clostridium botulinum – Blocks ACh release → flaccid paralysis
• E. coli (ETEC) – Heat-labile toxin ↑ cAMP, Heat-stable toxin ↑ cGMP → diarrhea
• Vibrio cholerae – Cholera toxin activates Gs protein → watery diarrhea
• Shigella – Shiga toxin inactivates 60S ribosome → dysentery

DNA vs RNA Viruses – Key Differences

Feature	DNA Viruses	RNA Viruses
Genome type	Double-stranded (except Parvo)	Single-stranded (except Reo)
Location of replication	Nucleus (except Pox)	Cytoplasm (except Retro, Influenza)
Examples	Herpes, Hep B, Adeno, Parvo, Pox	Influenza, HIV, HCV, Rabies, Dengue

Hepatitis Markers – Interpretation Made Easy

- HBsAg: Indicates active infection (acute or chronic)
- Anti-HBs: Indicates recovery or vaccination
- Anti-HBc IgM: Marker of acute infection
- Anti-HBc IgG: Past or chronic infection
- HBeAg: Active viral replication (infectivity marker)
- Anti-HBe: Lower infectivity

DNA Virus Families – Must Know

- Herpesviridae – HSV, VZV, CMV, EBV
- Hepadnaviridae – Hepatitis B virus
- Adenoviridae – Conjunctivitis, pharyngitis
- Papovaviridae – HPV, JC virus
- Poxviridae – Smallpox, Molluscum contagiosum (largest DNA virus)
- Parvoviridae – Parvovirus B19 (smallest DNA virus)

Fungi – Classification & Clinical Relevance

Type of Fungus	Form	Examples / Diseases
Yeasts	Unicellular	Candida albicans, Cryptococcus neoformans
Molds	Multicellular (hyphae)	Aspergillus, Mucor, Rhizopus
Dimorphic	Yeast in tissue, mold in environment	Histoplasma, Blastomyces, Coccidioides
Opportunistic	Affect immunocompromised	Candida, Aspergillus, Mucor, Cryptococcus

Fungal Stains – Diagnostic Utility

- KOH mount – Initial screening for fungi (hair, nail, skin)
- India ink – Cryptococcus neoformans (capsule visualization)
- PAS stain – Highlights fungal cell wall (positive in Candida, Aspergillus)

• GMS (Gomori Methenamine Silver) – Black staining of fungal elements
• Calcofluor white – Fluorescent stain binding fungal cell wall chitin

Parasitology – Important Helminths & Protozoa

• Plasmodium spp. – Malaria (falciparum most severe)
• Entamoeba histolytica – Amoebic dysentery, liver abscess
• Giardia lamblia – Fatty diarrhea (steatorrhea), fecal-oral spread
• Ascaris lumbricoides – Intestinal obstruction
• Taenia solium – Pork tapeworm, causes cysticercosis
• Wuchereria bancrofti – Filariasis, elephantiasis
• Echinococcus granulosus – Hydatid cyst (liver)

www.ingramcontent.com/pod-product-compliance
Ingram Content Group UK Ltd.
Pitfield, Milton Keynes, MK11 3LW, UK
UKHW061539190726
13845UKWH00031B/1124

9 789334 283570